# NEUROLOGY RECALL
## 2ND EDITION

D1153550

# NEUROLOGY RECALL

## 2ND EDITION

**JAMES Q. MILLER, M.D.**
Alumni Professor of Neurology
Department of Neurology
University of Virginia School of Medicine
Charlottesville, Virginia


**NATHAN B. FOUNTAIN, M.D.**
Associate Professor of Neurology
Department of Neurology
University of Virginia School of Medicine
Charlottesville, Virginia

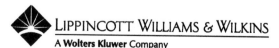

LIPPINCOTT WILLIAMS & WILKINS
A **Wolters Kluwer** Company

Philadelphia • Baltimore • New York • London
Buenos Aires • Hong Kong • Sydney • Tokyo

*Senior Acquisitions Editor:* Neil Marquardt
*Managing Editor:* Amy Oravec
*Marketing Manager:* Scott Lavine
*Production Editor:* Caroline Define
*Designer:* Risa Clow
*Compositor:* TechBooks
*Printer:* Malloy Inc.

351 West Camden Street
Baltimore, MD 21201

530 Walnut Street
Philadelphia, PA 19106

*Printed in the United States of America*

First Edition, 1997

**Library of Congress Cataloging-in-Publication Data**

CIP data has been applied for and is available from the Library of Congress.

To purchase additional copies of this book, call our customer service department at
**(800) 638-3030** or fax orders to **(301) 824-7390.** International customers should
call **(301) 714-2324.**

***Visit Lippincott Williams & Wilkins on the Internet: http://www.LWW.com.***
Lippincott Williams & Wilkins customer service representatives are available from
8:30 am to 6:00 pm, EST.

02 03 04 05 06
1 2 3 4 5 6 7 8 9 10

# Dedication

This book is dedicated to the students we have taught and from whom we have learned.

# RECALL SERIES EDITOR

**LORNE H. BLACKBOURNE, M.D.**
General Surgeon
Major, Medical Corps
United States Army
Fort Eustis, Virginia

# Contents

## SECTION IV
## OTHER IMPORTANT NEUROLOGIC CONDITIONS

## SECTION V
## PEDIATRIC NEUROLOGY

## SECTION VI
## DIAGNOSTIC PROCEDURES IN NEUROLOGY

## LIST OF TABLES

## DIAGRAMS FOR REFERENCES

# Contributors

The following physicians in the Department of Neurology contributed to or reviewed portions of the first edition of this book as faculty:

James P. Bennett, Jr., M.D., Ph.D.
Thomas P. Bleck, M.D.
Edward H. Bertram, M.D.
H. Robert Brashear, M.D.
David G. Brock, M.D.
Fritz E. Dreifuss, M.B., FRCP, FRACP
E. Clarke Haley, M.D.
George R. Hanna, M.D.

Madaline B. Harrison, M.D.
Vern C. Juel, M.D.
Ivan S. Login, M.D.
James Q. Miller, M.D.
W. Davis Parker, Jr., M.D.
Lawrence H. Phillips, II, M.D.
Joel M. Trugman, M.D.
G. Frederick Wooten, Jr., M.D.

The following physicians in the Department of Neurology contributed to and reviewed portions of the first edition of this book as housestaff:

Robert F. Armstrong, M.D.
W. Scott Bridges, M.D.
Alton E. Bryant, M.D.
Cherylee W.J. Chang, M.D.
William B. Dawson, M.D.
Gwendolyn F. Ford, M.D.
Nathan B. Fountain, M.D.
William T. Garrett, M.D.
Mitzi K. Hemstreet, M.D., Ph.D.
Steven F. Karner, M.D.
Kenneth V. Leone, M.D.
Barnett R. Nathan, M.D.

Troy A. Payne, M.D.
Javier J. Provencio, M.D.
Mark S. Quigg, M.D.
Christopher S. Scherer, M.D.
Elaine J. Skalabrin, M.D.
Robb M. Snider, M.D.
Nina J. Solenski, M.D.
J. Scott Story, M.D.
Russell H. Swerdlow, M.D.
Jay A. Van Gerpen, M.D.
Alan S. Zacharias, M.D.

The following physicians also contributed to the first edition of this book:

Maurice H. Lipper, MBChB, FACR, Associate Professor of Radiology
B. Todd Sitzman, M.D., M.P.H., Resident in Anesthesiology

Special contributions to the second edition of *Neurology Recall* were made by:

Vern C. Juel, M.D.
Mark S. Quigg, M.D.
Russell H. Swerdlow, M.D.
Cynthia Westley, R.N, M.S.N., A.N.Pc.
Thomas Bleck, Ph.D., M.D.

# Foreword

This second edition of *Neurology Recall* serves to improve and update the First Edition published in 1997. Drs. Fountain and Miller, with a little help from their friends, have added and re-formatted numerous illustrations, updated material based on recent advances in diagnosis and treatment of neurologic diseases, and added new sections on neurogenetics, ethics, bioterrorism, and child neurology.

The lasting utility of this book, however, remains embodied in the unique approach that Dr. Miller has evolved over a 45-year neurologic career aimed at introducing the key concepts of clinical neurology to students. The focus on common, urgent, and treatable symptoms is a time-honored and successful approach at both the undergraduate and graduate levels.

*Neurology Recall* continues to provide an effective framework whereby future generations of medical students and generalist physicians can learn the practical, useful principles of clinical neurology.

G. Frederick Wooten, M.D.
Chair and Mary Anderson Harrison Professor of Neurology
University of Virginia School of Medicine

# Preface

This book provides a user-friendly format to learn and review the essential aspects of clinical neurology. Written with the needs of the medical student in mind, it will also serve to guide the beginning house officer and physicians in non-neurologic fields who seek a current overview.

The basic information that underlies diagnosis and management of disease of the nervous system is emphasized. As with the first edition of *Neurology Recall*, this second edition uses a question and answer format covering both the original materiel and much new information now available to improve neurologic diagnosis and treatment; the pharmacotherapies of epilepsy, Parkinson's disease, multiple sclerosis, and headache are examples. There are several new features designed particularly to aid the student, including a table summarizing current neurogenetic information, an expanded set of "neuroanatomic road maps" to explain the routes by which a nerve impulse gets from here to there, and expanded illustrations of neuroimages and electrodiagnostic tests.

Many new areas of importance have been added, including the basic elements of ethics in the care of neurologic patients and of bioterrorism from a neurologic perspective.

# Section 1

Introduction and
Background
Information

# 1     Introduction

## HOW THIS BOOK IS DIFFERENT FROM OTHER BOOKS

Academic learning includes reading, listening to, understanding, and memorizing information. Didactic textbooks provide detailed information and a conceptual framework for understanding; however, because textbooks are so expansive, they may not clearly indicate what information is most important to understand and memorize. *Neurology Recall* is intended to aid memorization by pointing out important facts and helping you understand them.

*Neurology Recall* uses several methods to help you learn and memorize. First, the book emphasizes information that is considered important or standard knowledge. Second, the question-and-answer format focuses your attention on the most important information, allowing you to think about a problem independent from its context in a textbook and then solidify the facts in your memory. Third, the material is stated simplistically and organized in a fashion suited for systematic problem solving. Fourth, there are mnemonics and Do-It-Yourself diagrams to help you solve problems and understand answers.

## HOW THIS BOOK IS ORGANIZED

All of the chapters in a section are structured in a similar sequence. Sometimes, the structure is explicit. For example, Chapter 4, Differential Diagnosis of Common Problems, provides a table of diagnoses for each problem. The tables are structured in a specific format, rather than a laundry list of diagnoses. Therefore, if you memorize the structure of the table, it will help you recall the individual diseases. Furthermore, this method of listing the differential diagnoses provides a framework that allows you to add additional diagnoses not covered in this book. For example, there are 22 diseases listed as causes of myopathy, but they are grouped into only three categories: inflammatory myopathies, noninflammatory myopathies, and muscular dystrophies. By categorizing the diseases, you can remember the most important diseases for each category or subdivide the categories. For example, inflammatory myopathies can be divided into infectious and noninfectious inflammatory myopathies.

Sometimes, the structure is implicit. For example, the questions in each chapter of Section II, Common Neurologic Conditions, are organized in a similar fashion so that you can anticipate the general order of questions. For each disease, there are questions about the essential factors that define a disease: **etiology** and **epidemiology, pathology** and **pathogenesis, symptoms** and **signs, diagnostic tests, differential diagnosis,** and **treatment** and **prognosis.** For each disease, at least one important fact about each of these six factors should be recalled by the student.

## Organization of Questions

The questions are organized for Socratic teaching. You should start at the beginning of a section and proceed through it to the end. The first question in a chapter usually addresses a general issue and each following question builds on the preceding question. More detail is elicited with each subsequent question. The questions are designed not to give away too much information. Instead, the questions provide clues and hints, so that the reader may recall the answers to succeeding questions even if he did not know the answer to the original question. Information that is too detailed for students to volunteer but helpful for understanding the material has been added to the answer. However, we do not necessarily expect the reader to know this additional information. For example, a question may ask, "What is the inheritance pattern of Wilson's disease?" The answer is "Autosomal recessive. The defect is on chromosome 13." It is reasonable to expect students to know the mode of inheritance, but they are probably not expected to know which chromosome contains the abnormality.

## HOW TO USE THIS BOOK

This book complements a standard neurology textbook—it does not replace it. First read the relevant portions of a neurology textbook, so that you understand the rationale for approaching neurologic problems in a specific manner. After you have read about a chapter in a standard textbook, use the relevant sections of this book to test yourself and to discern the most important information. By covering the answers on the right side of the page with the bookmark, you can attempt to answer the question to evaluate your understanding of the information.

Alternatively, you may use this book to learn the important aspects of a disease. For example, if a fellow student admits a patient with an unfamiliar disease, you may study the relevant sections of this book to learn the basics about that disease. Finally, you may use this book to quiz yourself or to prepare for a neurology clerkship test. This book is probably most useful in small quantities; you can use it while waiting for rounds to begin or waiting for the bus. Keep the book with you and use it in spare minutes either alone or with fellow students, playing "neurojeopardy" with one another.

## APPROACHING NEUROLOGY PATIENTS USING THE "NEUROLOGIC FORMULATION"

Neurology diagnosis uses symptoms and signs to localize the site of a lesion and then uses the location to help determine the likely diagnosis. Therefore, an entire section of this book is devoted to neuroanatomy, which is essential to understanding localization.

The **neurologic formulation** is a structured approach to neurologic problems and is *always* used on neurology rounds during a patient assessment. It is analogous to the "impression" used during rounds in other clerkships. The formulation conveys a significant amount of information in a brief statement. It should contain enough detail for the listener or reader to accurately diagnose the condition, but it should not be a reiteration of the complete history. Summation and correlation are paramount to keeping the audience's attention. The formulation should be no more than three or four sentences. The following method is almost universally applicable.

## EXAMPLE OF A FORMULATION

Patient X is a 63-year-old right-handed woman with significant past medical history (PMH) of diabetes and hyperlipidemia who presents with acute word-finding difficulty and right-sided weakness. On examination she has nonfluent aphasia referable to the left frontal cortex and right hemiparesis involving the lower face, arm, and leg, with upper motor neuron signs referable to the corticobulbar and corticospinal tracts subserving the right side of the body. This is consistent with a single lesion in the left frontal cortex. The most likely diagnosis is ischemic infarction in the distribution of the left middle cerebral artery (MCA) from artery-to-artery embolus, but the differential diagnosis (DDx) includes left MCA thrombosis, cardiogenic embolus, and left frontal hemorrhage.

## FILL-IN-THE-BLANK FORMULATION

Patient _____ is a _____ year-old **right/left**-handed **man/woman** with significant PMH of _____ , _____, _____ who presents with _____ . On examination there is _____ referable to _____ , and _____ referable to _____ . This is consistent with a lesion(s) at _____ . The most likely diagnosis is _____ , but the DDx includes _____ , _____ , and _____ .

The formulation follows a specific order:

1. The **identifying data** always contains the patient's age, sex, race, and usually handedness. However, if handedness and race are not relevant, they may be omitted.
2. Include only the **PMH** significant to the current problem in your formulation, even if the patient has other important medical conditions or a history of severe medical illness (e.g., traumatic splenectomy). These other medical conditions should be omitted in the formulation unless it helps develop the DDx.
3. A **statement of the problem** is not necessarily the chief complaint. Instead, it is a summary of your interpretation of the patient's main problem. For example, the chief complaint may be that the patient has difficulty speaking, which is not very specific in developing the DDx. Phrase it in more specific neurologic diagnostic terminology. For example, state that the patient has "slurred speech" or "word-finding difficulty."
4. The **physical examination findings** are a summary of the relevant findings, not a complete detail, of the physical examination. For example, stating that the patient has "right hemiparesis with upper motor neuron signs" is more concise than stating he has "right-sided weakness, hyperreflexia, upgoing toe, etc." Traditionally, physical findings are omitted from the formulation and only a statement of their localization is used. However, in

the best formulation, you should summarize the physical findings, identify the involved pathways and the highest level of the nervous system affected, and then state the location where all of these coincide, or "cross." This location is where a single lesion is probably located. Some diseases are multifocal or generalized, and this should be your conclusion in the formulation.

5. Stating the most likely **diagnosis** commits you to a single diagnosis. If the statements in your formulation are logical, the audience will come to the same conclusion. However, a DDx is usually appropriate in a formulation, because the diagnosis is almost never absolutely certain. The DDx may be based on location of the lesion (i.e., anatomic DDx) or etiology of the lesion (i.e., congenital/genetic, toxic/metabolic, infectious, neoplastic, traumatic, autoimmune). An etiologic DDx is most specific and useful.

## THE NEUROLOGY CLERKSHIP

## STUDYING FOR THE NEUROLOGY CLERKSHIP

Your study objectives for the neurology clerkship should include the following goals.

**Learn to localize.** Many nervous system diseases are best understood if they are localized to a point in the nervous system. Simplistically, neurologic diseases localize to one of three locations:

1. **One location in the nervous system**, such as a bullet wound of the cerebellum, or **multiple individual locations,** such as the plaques of multiple sclerosis
2. The **entire nervous system,** as occurs in hypoglycemia
3. The **components of a neurologic subsystem**, as occurs in a motor neuron disease, such as amyotrophic lateral sclerosis

**Approaching patients.** Use the following three questions to approach patients:

1. Is there disease of the nervous system?
2. Where is it?
3. What can it be?

You will understand neurologic disorders better if you base them in clinical neuroanatomy and applied neurophysiology. Skim Section I, Introduction and Clinically Useful Neuroanatomy, so you know its contents and can refer back when necessary.

**Analyze the disease.** Analyze the disease not only by anatomic location but also by course of the illness. These two features, derived from the history and the physical examination, are the best indicators of appropriate diagnostic and management options. When you become a neurologic detective and analyze the clues properly, each patient becomes a mystery to solve and help. The analysis is largely a clinical task that depends on your eyes and ears as well as the physical examination and sophisticated diagnostic aids. However, despite the helpfulness of CT scans and MRIs, neurologic diagnosis and care largely depend on the physician's examination skills and analytical abilities.

**Identify instructive patients.** Concentrate on two or three patients each day whom you are caring for or about whom your team is talking. Read about their particular disease in a standard neurology text. With this approach, you will understand and remember what you have observed during your neurology clerkship.

Your time is limited in a neurology clerkship. Nevertheless, there are three goals to accomplish: you should understand your patients, learn about the diseases encountered by other members of your team, and learn essentials of the core nervous system diseases that have not been covered in your medical school experiences. To accomplish these three goals, a student should focus on those conditions that are common, urgent, treatable, illustrative of important biologic principles, or those that point to improved understanding.

## EXAMINATION EQUIPMENT: WHAT YOU SHOULD CARRY WITH YOU OR BE ABLE TO ACCESS

**Essential:**
    Bright penlight
    Reflex hammer
    Stethoscope
    Ophthalmo/otoscope
**Helpful:**
    128 cps tuning fork
    Safety pins
    Cotton wisp or tissue
    Vision near card
    Piece of transparent red plastic for diplopia or (Frenzel lens)
    Tape measure (babies)
**Helpful, But Not Essential:**
    Vial of cold or warm water
    Stoppered vials of coffee/cinnamon
    Stoppered vials of sugar/salt
    Bright plastic toy car (children)
    Small hand bell (babies)

## PRESENTING ON NEUROLOGIC ROUNDS

Whether you are in an ambulatory or in-patient setting, remember the **four Cs:** Be **cooperative, considerate, cleanly dressed** (your patients deserve it), and **concise.** It is appropriate to refer to notes but not to read them; it is better to omit information and be asked about it than to cover everything in a boring tone.

A word about dress: Arrive in a white coat, wearing a tie if you are a man, and then judge what to wear based on your team or service's attire. Dress varies greatly among locales, and it is an item of less importance once you get to know your patients and attendings. Most doctors dress in a manner that easily identifies themselves as physicians to patients and visitors. Many may wear a white coat or scrub suit. Your goal is to make your patients and colleagues comfortable in your presence.

## ORGANIZING YOUR PRESENTATION

State the patient's age, chief complaint, duration of complaint, and course of illness. Mention any history of a neurologic problem before onset of the present illness, because many neurologic conditions are chronic and diagnosis demands understanding the patient's previous neurologic health. Include all aspects of the history that point toward a diagnosis. Omit extraneous facts that you think are irrelevant to understanding your patient's current condition. Relate the patient's physical findings as they were at the time of admission or onset of the present illness. Include subsequent alterations in physical findings as part of the course of the illness if they are relevant. Also include results of laboratory and imaging studies as part of the course of the illness. Never begin your presentation stating that the patient is admitted because of a CT scan, etc. Also, it is a neurologic nicety to indicate the patient's handedness as part of the physical findings.

### Presenting the Physical Findings

A good presentation includes everything that the audience needs to know, and nothing else. Improve your presentations by analyzing your contemporaries. Ideally, you should only list normal physical findings if needed to prevent misinformation or ambiguity; otherwise, simply state the examination is normal. List the physical findings in sequence from top to bottom.

### General Physical Examination

1. Vital signs
2. Relevant physical findings (Normal findings do not need to be listed individually)

### Neurologic Examination

The basic neurologic examination is straightforward and logically organized. It is most useful to perform the components in the same manner on all patients. The five parts of a basic neurologic examination are listed below. To avoid becoming confused or forgetting portions, complete one part before continuing on to the next. Use the hints in parentheses to help organize each portion. Performing a "basic" examination on a patient without physical findings should take no more than 10 minutes once you are familiar with the procedure.

Mental Status:

Orientation, speech, memory, praxis
Mini-mental status examination (MMSE) if appropriate

Cranial Nerves:

*(start at the top of the face with the eyes and work to the bottom, which corresponds numerically with starting at CN II and working inferiorly)*

| (II) | Visual acuity, visual fields (VF) |
| (III, IV, VI) | Extraocular muscles (EOM) pupils, fundus (*examine after above because of the brightness of the light*) |
| (V) | Facial sensation, lateral jaw movement |
| (VII) | Facial symmetry, strength |
| (VIII) | Auditory acuity |
| (IX, X) | Palate symmetry and strength |
| (XI) | Sternocleidomastoid strength |
| (XII) | Tongue protrusion |

## Motor:

*(work from proximal to distal; both arms, then both legs)*
Bulk, tone, and strength
Deep tendon reflexes (DTRs)
Pathologic reflexes (Babinski, Hoffman)

## Sensory:

pinprick, temperature, light touch *(test at least one spinothalamic tract modality)*
proprioception, vibration *(test at least one dorsal column pathway modality)*

## Coordination:

Upper extremity—finger to nose, rapid alternating movements
Lower extremity—heel-to-knee-to-shin, parallel and heel-to-toe gait, Romberg

## HELPFUL ONLINE SITES

American Academy of Neurology
   www.neurology.org
American Neurological Association
   www.aneuroa.org
End of life issues
   www.partnershipforcaring.org
Genetic basis of diseases
   www.OMIM
Merck Manual
   www.merck.com/pubs/mmanual/section14/sec14.html
Neurological examination
   www.medinfo.ufl.edu/year1/bcs/clist/neuro.html
Neuropathology images
   www-medlib.med.utah.edu/WebPath/webpath/html

# 2

# Common Abbreviations

Abbreviations are useful for medical records, and there are a lot of them in neurology. Before you use an abbreviation, make sure your reader will understand it; it is difficult to try to guess what someone else means in a written record. For example, what does PND mean? Paroxysmal nocturnal dyspnea or postnasal drip?

## ABBREVIATIONS

| | |
|---|---|
| **5-HT** | Five hydroxytryptophan |
| **ā** | Before |
| **ACA** | Anterior cerebral artery |
| **ACh** | Acetylcholine |
| **AED** | Antiepileptic drug |
| **ALS** | Amyotrophic lateral sclerosis |
| **ANA** | Antinuclear antibody |
| **APD** | Afferent pupillary defect |
| **ASA** | Acetylsalicylic acid (aspirin) |
| **AVM** | Arteriovenous malformation |
| **BAEP** | Brain stem auditory-evoked potential |
| **BAER** | Brain stem auditory-evoked response (same as BAEP) |
| **BG** | Basal ganglia |
| **BP** | Blood pressure |
| **c̄** | With |
| **CA** | Cancer |

| | |
|---|---|
| **CABG** | Coronary artery bypass graft |
| **CBZ** | Carbamazepine |
| **CIDP** | Chronic inflammatory demyelinating polyneuropathy |
| **CMG** | Cystometrogram |
| **CMT** | Charcot-Marie-Tooth disease |
| **CP** | Cerebral palsy or closing pressure |
| **CPA** | Cerebellopontine angle |
| **CPK** | Creatine phosphokinase |
| **CPS** | Complex partial seizure |
| **CSF** | Cerebrospinal fluid |
| **CT (CAT SCAN)** | Computerized axial tomography |
| **CTS** | Carpal tunnel syndrome |
| **CVA** | Cerebrovascular attack |
| **CXR** | Chest radiograph |
| **DDx** | Differential diagnosis |
| **DJD** | Degenerative joint disease |
| **DP** | Dorsalis pedis |
| **DPH** | Diphenylhydantoin (phenytoin) |
| **DTR** | Deep tendon reflex |
| **Dx** | Diagnosis |
| **EEG** | Electroencephalogram |
| **EMG** | Electromyogram |
| **EOM** | Extra ocular movements |
| **ESR** | Erythrocyte sedimentation rate |

| | |
|---|---|
| **ETOH** | Ethyl alcohol |
| **F to N** | Finger to nose |
| **FSH** | Facio-scapulo-humeral muscular dystrophy |
| **GBS** | Guillain-Barré syndrome |
| **GTC** | Generalized tonic clonic seizure |
| **H to S** | Heel to shin |
| **HA** | Headache |
| **HC** | Head circumference |
| **HNP** | Herniated nucleus pulposus |
| **HSMN** | Hereditary sensorimotor neuropathy |
| **HTN** | Hypertension |
| **ICH** | Intracerebral hemorrhage |
| **ICP** | Intracranial pressure |
| **INO** | Internuclear ophthalmoplegia |
| **LBP** | Low back pain |
| **LE** | Lower extremity |
| **LMN** | Lower motor neuron |
| **LP** | Lumbar puncture |
| **MBP** | Myelin basic protein |
| **MCA** | Middle cerebral artery |
| **MD** | Muscular dystrophy |
| **MLF** | Medial longitudinal fasciculus |
| **MPTP** | Methyl-phenyl-tetrahydropyridine |
| **MR** | Mental retardation |

| | |
|---|---|
| **MRA** | Magnetic resonance angiogram |
| **MRI** | Magnetic resonance image |
| **MRS** | Magnetic resonance spectroscopy |
| **MS** | Multiple sclerosis |
| **NCS** | Nerve conduction study |
| **NCSE** | Nonconvulsive status epilepticus |
| **NCV** | Nerve conduction velocity |
| **NICE** | Noninvasive carotid evaluation |
| **NMJ** | Neuromuscular junction |
| **NPH** | Normal pressure hydrocephalus |
| **NPO** | Nothing by mouth (per os) |
| **NS** | Normal saline |
| **OCBs** | Oligoclonal bands |
| **OP** | Opening pressure |
| **OPCA** | Olivopontocerebellar atrophy |
| **OT** | Occupational therapy |
| **p̄** | After |
| **Pb** | Phenobarbital |
| **PCA** | Posterior cerebral artery |
| **PD** | Parkinson's disease |
| **PE** | Pulmonary embolism |
| **PERRLA** | Pupils equal round and reactive to light and accommodation |
| **PET** | Positron emission tomography |
| **PICA** | Posterior inferior cerebellar artery |

| | |
|---|---|
| **PLEDS** | Periodic lateralizing epileptiform discharges |
| **PML** | Progressive multifocal leukoencephalopathy |
| **prn** | As needed |
| **PSP** | Progressive supranuclear palsy |
| **PT** | Physical therapy |
| **PT** | Prothrombin time |
| **qod** | Every other day |
| **qd** | Every day |
| **qid** | Four times per day |
| **RAM** | Rapid alternating movements |
| **REM** | Rapid eye movement |
| **RF** | Rheumatoid factor |
| **RF** | Reticular formation |
| **ROM** | Range of motion |
| **SAH** | Subarachnoid hemorrhage |
| **SCM** | Sternocleidomastoid |
| **SOB** | Shortness of breath |
| **SPECT** | Single photon emission computerized tomography |
| **SSEP** | Somatosensory-evoked potentials |
| **SSPE** | Subacute sclerosing panencephalitis |
| **STAT** | Immediately |
| **TCA** | Tricyclic antidepressant |
| **TEE** | Transesophageal echocardiography |

| | |
|---|---|
| **TIA** | Transient ischemic attack |
| **TLE** | Temporal lobe epilepsy |
| **TMJ** | Temporomandibular joint |
| **UBOs** | Unidentified bright objects |
| **UE** | Upper extremity |
| **UMN** | Upper motor neuron |
| **UTI** | Urinary tract infection |
| **VDRL** | Venereal Disease Research Laboratory (test) |
| **VEP** | Visual evoked potential |
| **VFFC** | Visual fields full to confrontation |
| **VPA** | Valproic acid |
| **VPS** | Ventriculoperitoneal shunt |
| **WNL** | Within normal limits |
| $\bar{x}$ | Except |

# 3      Neuroanatomy

## CLINICAL NEUROANATOMIC PEARLS

**Pupil size**
**See also p. 52–55**

Pupil size is an interplay between parasympathetic and sympathetic stimuli. Parasympathetic stimuli originate in cranial nerve (CN) III of the midbrain and cause pupilloconstriction. They arrive via the oculomotor nerve. Sympathetic stimuli, contributing to pupillodilation, originate in the hypothalamus and descend to cord level T-1 before emerging from the neuraxis. Then, they ascend to the eye in the sympathetic nerve, accompanying the common and internal carotid arteries.

## NEUROANATOMIC ROAD MAP

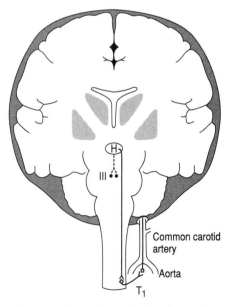

Parasympathetic and sympathetic pathways from hypothalamus (H) to pupil:
     ----- parasympathetic
     —— sympathetic

**Pupillary light reflex**
**See also p. 52–55**

The pupillary light reflex begins with illumination of the retina. Nerve impulses pass directly back through the optic nerve, chiasm, tract, and lateral geniculate without synapse to nuclei in the roof of the midbrain, the pretectal area. These neurons innervate both third-nerve nuclei, whose parasympathetic discharge causes bilateral pupilloconstriction in response to unilateral eye illumination. (See figure below and figures on facing page.)

## NEUROANATOMIC ROAD MAP

Path from retina to Edinger-Westphal component of CN III nucleus in midbrain

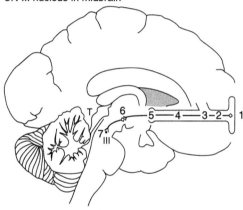

1 - Retina
2 - Optic nerve
3 - Chiasm
4 - Optic tract
5 - Lateral geniculate body
6 - Pretectal nuclei
7 - Nucleus CN III
T - Tectum

Location of pretectal area of brainstem on coronal
and sagittal section

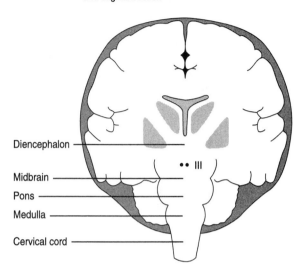

Diencephalon

Midbrain

Pons

Medulla

Cervical cord

•• III

Level of Pretectal Area of Brainstem

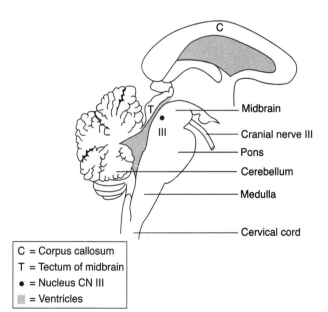

C

T

III

Midbrain

Cranial nerve III

Pons

Cerebellum

Medulla

Cervical cord

C = Corpus callosum
T = Tectum of midbrain
• = Nucleus CN III
▨ = Ventricles

**Visual pathway**
**See also p. 52**

The visual pathway is topographically highly organized. Because it is a major front-to-back tract, it is useful in localizing intracranial lesions. To understand this pathway, recall that the lens reverses light rays, so that the lower retina sees the upper visual world, and the left side of the retina sees the right visual world. Because the right and left eye visual fields overlap largely, the right side of the visual world is seen by the left side of both retinas simultaneously.

**Hemianopia and**
**quadrantanopia**

These two defects depend on the organization of the pathways from retinas to occipital cortex in both hemispheres. A left-pathway lesion blinds both left retinas, which see the right visual world, and causes a **right homonymous hemianopia.** The visual pathway also conducts images seen by the lower part of the retina, back to the inferior occipital cortex. A lesion of only the inferior portion of the left visual pathway would blind only the left inferior portion of the retinas and cause a **right superior quadrantanopia.**

## NEUROANATOMIC ROAD MAP

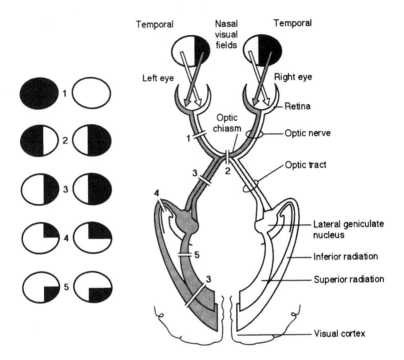

(Adapted with permission from Fix JD: *High-Yield Neuroanatomy.* Baltimore, Williams & Wilkins, 1995, p 74.)

**Vertical gaze**
**See also p. 55–58**

Vertical gaze depends on coordinated contractions of extraocular muscles innervated by CN III and CN IV. These nuclei are innervated by a gaze center in the rostral midbrain. Impairment of bilateral vertical gaze suggests a lesion in the roof of the midbrain (the tectum). (See figure on facing page.)

**Horizontal gaze**
**See also p. 55–58**

Conjugate horizontal gaze requires coordinated contractions of one lateral rectus muscle (CN VI) and the medial rectus muscle of the opposite eye (CN III). (See figure on facing page.) Voluntary horizontal conjugate gaze originates in the frontal cortex, where the frontal gaze center projects down to the contralateral pons. Involuntary horizontal conjugate gaze, as in horizontal nystagmus, is a response to vestibular input. Both cortical voluntary and vestibular involuntary impulses for conjugate horizontal gaze play upon the pontine center for lateral gaze. This functional center has several names, including the paramedian pontine reticular formation (PPRF) and the para-abducens nucleus. The center for horizontal or lateral gaze is composed of neurons intermingled with those of the abducens nucleus and adjacent areas of the pons. They innervate the ipsilateral CN VI nucleus. They also innervate the contralateral CN III nucleus via axons that cross the midline and ascend to the midbrain in the myelinated median longitudinal fasciculus (MLF). Discharge of a horizontal gaze center permits simultaneous stimulation of the ipsilateral sixth and contralateral third nerves and, thereby, **conjugate horizontal gaze** toward the side of the discharging brain stem gaze center.

## NEUROANATOMIC ROAD MAPS

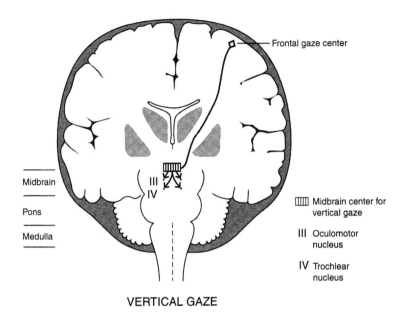

Frontal gaze center

Midbrain

Pons

Medulla

III  Oculomotor
IV

|||||| Midbrain center for
vertical gaze

III  Oculomotor
nucleus

IV  Trochlear
nucleus

**VERTICAL GAZE**

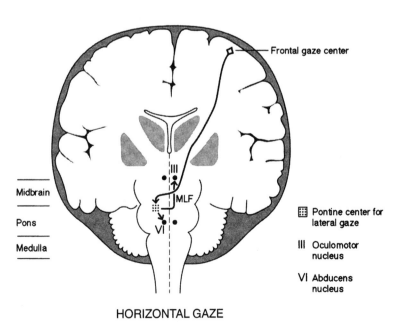

Frontal gaze center

Midbrain

Pons

Medulla

III

MLF

VI

▦ Pontine center for
lateral gaze

III  Oculomotor
nucleus

VI  Abducens
nucleus

**HORIZONTAL GAZE**

**Cerebellum**
**See also p. 77**

The cerebellum influences four aspects of neurologic function:
1. Synergy (i.e., coordination) from the cerebellar hemispheres
2. Posture from the vermis
3. Tone from the vermis
4. Vestibular function from the posterior vermis and flocculonodular lobes, which are also posterior

The **topographic localization** of the cerebellum is somewhat analogous to a butterfly: the midline vermis is the body of the butterfly and the hemispheres are the two wings. The vermis controls posture in the head, neck, and trunk, and each hemisphere controls coordination in the ipsilateral limb via the cerebellar double cross. The inferior posterior cerebellar vermis (i.e., the flocculonodular lobe) interacts with the vestibular system.

The **cerebellar double cross** is a pathway that leaves a cerebellar hemisphere through the superior cerebellar peduncle, decussates to the contralateral thalamus, and projects to that motor cortex. This cortex is now contralateral to the side of cerebellar origin. Upper motor neuron fibers originate here and descend via the pyramidal tract to decussate in the medulla and then innervate lower motor neurons ipsilateral to the originating cerebellar impulses. Therefore, cerebellar signs are ipsilateral to the involved cerebellar hemisphere.

## NEUROANATOMIC ROAD MAP

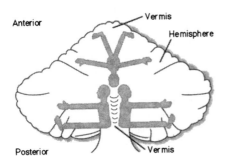

Anterior
Vermis
Hemisphere
Posterior
Vermis

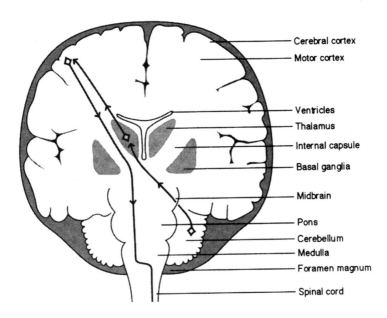

Cerebral cortex
Motor cortex
Ventricles
Thalamus
Internal capsule
Basal ganglia
Midbrain
Pons
Cerebellum
Medulla
Foramen magnum
Spinal cord

**Hearing**
See also p. 61

Impulses arrive over the auditory division of CN VIII. They almost immediately are distributed bilaterally on reaching the medulla and ascend bilaterally to both temporal lobes. Their routes include the cochlear nuclei and the trapezoid body in the medulla, the lateral lemnisci in the pons and midbrain, the medial geniculate nuclei in the diencephalon, and the temporal lobes. Because of the bilaterality of ascending pathways, there is no central nervous system cause for unilateral deafness once fibers leave the cochlear nuclei. Unilateral deafness usually is caused by disease in the cochlea of the inner ear in the temporal bone or in the eighth nerve itself. These processes often cause tinnitus and usually involve the vestibular receptors. Unilateral deafness, tinnitus, and vertigo often coexist, as in Ménière's syndrome.

## NEUROANATOMIC ROAD MAP

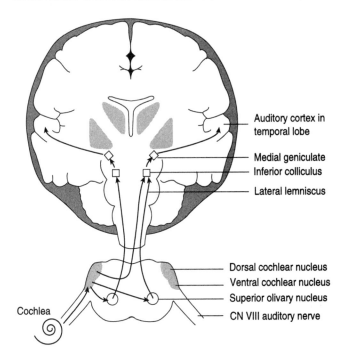

Auditory cortex in temporal lobe

Medial geniculate
Inferior colliculus

Lateral lemniscus

Dorsal cochlear nucleus
Ventral cochlear nucleus
Superior olivary nucleus
CN VIII auditory nerve

Cochlea

**Taste**
See also p. 60–61

Taste from the posterior tongue is conveyed centrally by the vagus and glossopharyngeal nerves. Taste from the anterior two thirds of the tongue travels in the lingual branch of the mandibular division of the trigeminal nerve (CN V$_3$) to the base of the tongue and then travels over the chorda tympani to the geniculate ganglion of the facial nerve (CN VII) in the facial canal. At this location, fibers turn sharply centrally to run inward to the nucleus of the solitary tract (i.e., nucleus solitarius) in the medulla. Therefore, taste fibers run opposite to emerging somatic motor facial nerve fibers that are also in the facial canal. Therefore, Bell's palsy (i.e., facial nerve palsy) may be associated with loss of taste on the anterior two thirds of the tongue if the nerve dysfunction is central to the geniculate ganglion.

**Eating**
See also p. 60–63

Eating is a complex neurologic endeavor that begins with biting and chewing, using the muscles of mastication (CN V). Food is then pushed backward by the tongue (CN XII) into the pharynx where the soft palate is raised (CN IX, CN X) to seal off the nasopharynx. Pharyngeal contraction (CN IX, CN X) forces food down into the esophagus while the glottis and larynx are closed (by action of CN IX and recurrent laryngeal of CN X). Peristalsis then conveys the bolus down the esophagus. Therefore, either upper motor neuron lesions or lower motor neuron deficits in CN IX, X, or XII can cause dysphagia.

## NEUROANATOMIC ROAD MAP

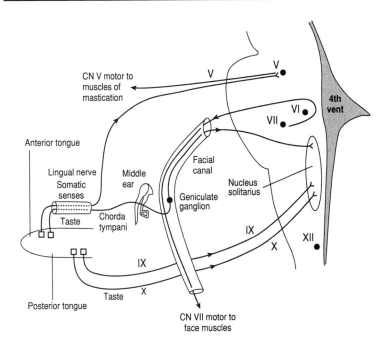

**Nystagmus**

Nystagmus is rhythmic jerking eye movement. It is either phasic or pendular. Phasic nystagmus, consisting of a slow and fast (i.e., saccadic) component, is a classic sign of vestibular dysfunction. Vertical nystagmus indicates brain stem disease. Horizontal and rotatory nystagmus can be either brain stem or peripheral in origin.

**Oculocephalic (cervico-ocular) reflex and caloric maneuvers**
See also p. 211–212, 218

This reflex, also known as the **doll's eye maneuver,** is an important clinical procedure that checks brain stem functioning in comatose patients. If the brain stem is functioning properly, rapid passive rotation of the patient's head in one direction stimulates the vestibular system so that the eyes deviate in the direction opposite to the head turn. Doll's eyes are not present in alert patients because visual fixation prevents this reflex. A more effective test is **cold water calorics,** which involves lavage of the tympanic membrane with 20 cc of ice water. In a patient with functioning vestibular pathways, it causes slow conjugate eye deviation toward the cold water. If the patient is awake, there will then be a fast movement (i.e., a saccade) in the opposite direction. It is conventional to name phasic nystagmus by the fast component. The mnemonic COWS—**c**old:**o**pposite; **w**arm:**s**ame— describes the direction of nystagmus in awake patients undergoing caloric testing. Remember, this mnemonic refers to the fast component, and some comatose patients only have slow eye deviation without the fast recovery phase.

## NEUROANATOMIC ROAD MAP

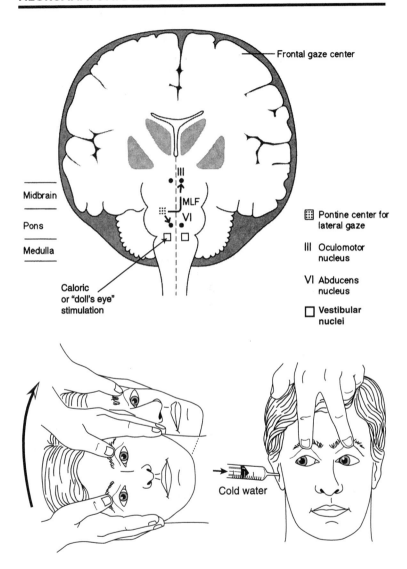

Frontal gaze center

Midbrain

Pons

Medulla

Caloric or "doll's eye" stimulation

⊞ Pontine center for lateral gaze

III Oculomotor nucleus

VI Abducens nucleus

☐ Vestibular nuclei

Cold water

**Somatic sensation**
**See also p. 70–74**

Somatic sensation arises in receptors throughout the body and is conveyed to the spinal cord in peripheral nerves. Sensation is conveyed to the brain across two primary spinal cord pathways. Pain and temperature impulses synapse in the spinal cord gray matter at or near the root of entry. They then cross the midline in front of the central canal of the cord and ascend in the contralateral *spinothalamic tract* in the white matter of the lateral spinal cord, continuing upward through the lateral medulla, pons, and midbrain to the thalamus. Then, thalamocortical pathways project to the sensory cortex in the parietal lobe. Position sensation, vibration, and deep pain enter the cord via posterior nerve roots, as do pain and temperature, but they ascend in the ipsilateral *posterior columns* to nuclei at the lowest end of the medulla. There, post-synaptic fibers cross and ascend in the middle of the medulla and then the lateral lemnisci of the pons and midbrain to the contralateral thalamus. Thalamocortical fibers then project to the parietal sensory cortex, opposite to the side of entry into the cord.

**Cortical sensation**

Cortical sensations include stereognosis, graphesthesia, and two-point discrimination. These sensations depend on integrity of the contralateral parietal cortex and may be lost in cortical lesions that leave other sensory modalities intact.

## NEUROANATOMIC ROAD MAPS

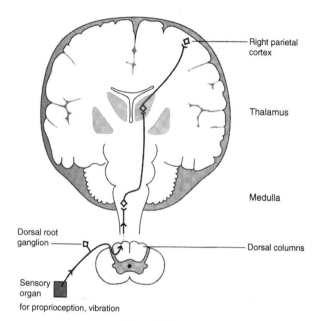

Right parietal cortex

Thalamus

Medulla

Dorsal root ganglion

Dorsal columns

Sensory organ

for proprioception, vibration

### Dorsal Column

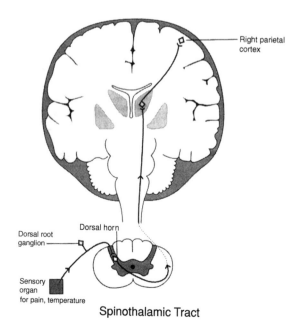

Right parietal cortex

Dorsal horn

Dorsal root ganglion

Sensory organ

for pain, temperature

### Spinothalamic Tract

**Urinary bladder**

The urinary bladder is a bag of smooth muscle which either stores or empties urine. Its function is an interplay of sympathetic and parasympathetic stimuli descending from a micturition center in the pons. *Storage* depends on sympathetic impulses via L2-L4 for contraction of the functional "internal sphincter" (muscle surrounding the outlet from bladder into urethra). *Emptying* accompanies bladder contraction due to parasympathetic impulses via S2,3,4.

Voluntary urination has three neurologic elements: a message from the frontal cortex to the micturition center in the pons which leads to sympathetic (L2,3,4) inhibition and parasympathetic (S2,3,4) discharge. Thirdly, simultaneous relaxation of voluntary muscles of the pelvic floor allows urine to pass through the functional "external sphincter."

## NEUROANATOMIC ROAD MAP

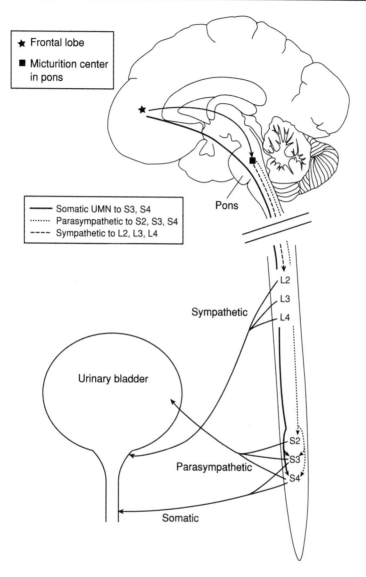

★ Frontal lobe

■ Micturition center
in pons

Pons

——— Somatic UMN to S3, S4
········· Parasympathetic to S2, S3, S4
– – – Sympathetic to L2, L3, L4

L2
L3
L4

Sympathetic

Urinary bladder

S2
S3
S4

Parasympathetic

Somatic

(Modified and reprinted with permission from Lerner A: *Little Black Book of Neurology*, 3rd ed. Mosby, 1995.)

# OVERVIEW OF NEUROANATOMY

## THE NERVOUS SYSTEM

| | |
|---|---|
| **What are the two major anatomic subdivisions of the nervous system?** | Central nervous system (CNS) and peripheral nervous system (PNS) |
| **Which originates inside bone and then emerges?** | Peripheral |
| **In what direction do most central neurologic pathways run?** | Longitudinal |
| **What are the three major longitudinal systems?** | 1. Somatic motor system<br>2. Somatic sensory system<br>3. Autonomic motor system |
| **What are two important horizontal systems that intersect the longitudinal systems?** | Visual pathways and peripheral nerves |
| **What is the name for an aggregate or clump of cell bodies in the nervous system that give rise to axons that run in a common pathway?** | Nucleus |
| **How do you localize a neurologic lesion?** | Determine which longitudinal and horizontal pathways and nuclei are affected, and then determine where they intersect. |
| **What are the two major anatomical components of the CNS?** | Brain and spinal cord |

## THE BRAIN IN THE SKULL

| | |
|---|---|
| **What are the two major compartments of the skull?** | Supratentorial and infratentorial |

**What is the tentorium?**

An infolding of posterior dura separating the cerebral hemispheres above from the cerebellum below

**What is the tentorial notch?**

An anterior opening in the tentorium allowing the brain stem from below to connect to the cerebrum above

**What is dura?**

A tough membrane overlying the brain. It is the inner periosteum of the cranium.

**What is arachnoid?**

A diaphanous membrane underlying the dura (and therefore another membrane overlying the brain)

**What is pia?**

A very thin membrane adherent to the surface of the cerebral cortex

**What are the leptomeninges?**

The pia and arachnoid together, enclosing a space between them

**What is the space between the arachnoid and pia called?**

Subarachnoid space

**What is in it?**

Cerebrospinal fluid (CSF) and bridging veins connecting the cortex to the arachnoid

**What comprises the meninges?**

Dura, arachnoid, and pia

**Considering the neuraxis as a layer cake, name the six layers from top to bottom.**

1. Cerebral hemispheres
2. Diencephalon (basal ganglia and thalamus)
3. Mesencephalon, or midbrain
4. Pons
5. Medulla
6. Spinal cord

**Which of these layers are intracranial?**

All of them except the spinal cord

**Which layer is in the tentorial notch?**

Midbrain

## CEREBROSPINAL FLUID

**Where is CSF made?**                    Choroid plexus

**Where is the choroid**                  In all four ventricles
**plexus?**

**Trace CSF from the lateral**            Lateral ventricle through interventricular
**ventricles to the fourth**              foramen to third ventricle through the
**ventricle.**                            aqueduct of Sylvius to fourth
                                          ventricle

**How does CSF exit from**                Through either the midline foramen of
**the fourth ventricle?**                 Magendie or the lateral foramina of
                                          Luschka (Remember: *m* for midline and
                                          Magendie and *l* for lateral and Luschka)

**Where does it go from**                 1. It enters the subarachnoid space (in
**there?**                                   cisterna magna), then
                                          2. It percolates up over hemispheres or
                                             down cord, and
                                          3. It is absorbed by arachnoid
                                             granulations

**What is the consequence**               Hydrocephalus of the lateral and third
**of obstruction of the**                 ventricles, which is a noncommunicating
**aqueduct of Sylvius?**                  hydrocephalus

**What is the consequence**               Hydrocephalus of all ventricles, which is a
**of obstruction in**                     communicating hydrocephalus
**subarachnoid space or**
**arachnoid granulations?**

**What is a cranial**                     Macrocephaly (i.e., large head size)
**consequence of neonatal**
**hydrocephalus?**

**What is the consequence of**            Increased intracranial pressure
**adult hydrocephalus?**

## CELLS OF THE NERVOUS SYSTEM

**What cell is the basic unit**           A neuron with its axon and dendrites
**of a neurologic tract?**

| | |
|---|---|
| **What cell's membranes constitute CNS myelin?** | Oligodendroglia |
| **What is the function of microglia?** | They act as phagocytes in CNS |
| **What cells line the ventricles?** | Ependyma (also called ependymal glia) |
| **What are the four types of glial cells?** | 1. Astroglia, or astrocytes<br>2. Oligodendroglia<br>3. Ependymoglia, or ependyma<br>4. Microglia |

## CRANIAL NERVES

| | |
|---|---|
| **How many cranial nerves are there?** | Twelve |
| **What makes a nerve a cranial nerve?** | It emerges through a cranial foramen. |
| **Which two cranial nerves are not composed of peripheral nervous tissue?** | Olfactory and optic nerves |
| **What is a mnemonic to name the cranial nerves?** | On Old Olympus' Towering Tops A Finn And German Viewed Some Hops |

| | | |
|---|---|---|
| **O**n | Olfactory | I |
| **O**ld | Optic | II |
| **O**lympus' | Oculomotor | III |
| **T**owering | Trochlear | IV |
| **T**ops | Trigeminal | V |
| **A** | Abducens | VI |
| **F**inn | Facial | VII |
| **A**nd | Auditory–vestibular | VIII |
| **G**erman | Glossopharyngeal | IX |
| **V**iewed | Vagus | X |
| **S**ome | Spinal accessory | XI |
| **H**ops | Hypoglossal | XII |

| | |
|---|---|
| **Which cranial nerves are exclusively sensory?** | CN I, CN II, CN VIII |

| | |
|---|---|
| **Which carry parasympathetic fibers?** | CN III to the pupil; CN VII to the lacrimal, submandibular, and sublingual glands; CN IX to the parotid gland; CN X to the viscera |
| **Which carry sympathetic fibers?** | None. The sympathetic nervous system is the thoracolumbar division of the autonomic nervous system. |
| **What are the three divisions of the trigeminal nerve (CN V)?** | 1. Ophthalmic ($V_1$), which receives sensation from above the angle of the eye<br>2. Maxillary ($V_2$), which receives sensation from the angle of eye down to angle of mouth<br>3. Mandibular ($V_3$), which receives sensation from below angle of mouth to angle of jaw |
| **What mnemonic identifies the foramen for the first, second, and third divisions of the trigeminal nerve?** | **S**tanding    **S**up. orb. fissure<br>**R**oom         **R**otundum<br>**O**nly          **O**vale |
| **What are the four muscles of mastication innervated by CN V?** | Temporalis, masseter, and two pterygoids |
| **What is the major function of the seventh cranial nerve?** | It innervates the muscles of facial expression |
| **What is a central seventh lesion?** | A unilateral UMN lesion disconnecting the motor cortex from the contra-lateral seventh nucleus in the pons |
| **What is its clinical manifestation?** | Paralysis of the lower face |

**Why can this patient still wrinkle his forehead and squeeze his eyes shut?**

The seventh-nerve (lower motor) neurons innervating the frontalis and orbicularis oculi muscles get a bilateral supply of corticobulbar (upper motor) neurons. Thus, a unilateral UMN lesion does not completely denervate them.

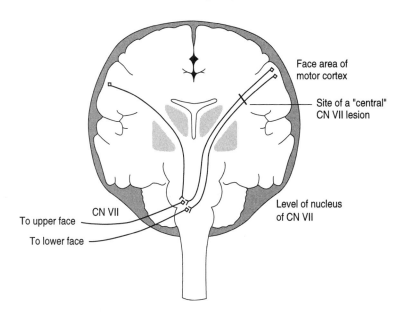

Face area of motor cortex

Site of a "central" CN VII lesion

Level of nucleus of CN VII

CN VII

To upper face

To lower face

**Which way does the palate elevate in a unilateral lesion of CN IX and X?**

Away from the damaged nerve

**Which way does sternocleidomastoid (CN XI) contraction pull the occiput?**

Forward, rotating the chin away from the contracting muscle

**Which way does the tongue protrude in unilateral weakness of the hypoglossal nerve (CN XII)?**

Toward the damaged nerve

**Select the appropriate foramen for each cranial nerve by drawing a
line from the nerve on the left to the foramen on the right.**

| Cranial Nerve | Foramina in Alphabetical Order |
|---|---|
| Olfactory nerve (I) | Cribriform plate |
| Optic nerve (II) | Facial canal and stylomastoid foramen |
| Oculomotor nerve (III) | Foramen ovale |
| Trochlear nerve (IV) | Foramen rotundum |
| Ophthalmic ($V_1$) | Hypoglossal foramen |
| Maxillary ($V_2$) | Internal acoustic meatus in petrous bone of skull |
| Mandibular ($V_3$) | Jugular foramen |
| Abducens nerve (VI) | Optic canal |
| Facial nerve (VII) | Superior orbital fissure |
| Cochlear/vestibular nerve (VIII) | |
| Glossopharyngeal (IX) | |
| Vagus nerve (X) | |
| Accessory nerve (XI) | |
| Hypoglossal nerve (XII) | |

**Answers**

| | |
|---|---|
| Olfactory nerve (I) | Cribriform plate |
| Optic nerve (II) | Optic canal |
| Oculomotor nerve (III) | Superior orbital fissure |
| Trochlear nerve (IV) | Superior orbital fissure |
| Ophthalmic ($V_1$) | Superior orbital fissure (**St**anding) |
| Maxillary ($V_2$) | Foramen rotundum (**R**oom) |
| Mandibular ($V_3$) | Foramen ovale (**O**nly) |
| Abducens nerve (VI) | Superior orbital fissure |
| Facial nerve (VII) | Facial canal and stylomastoid foramen |
| Cochlear/vestibular nerve (VIII) | Internal acoustic meatus in petrous bone of skull |
| Glossopharyngeal (IX) | Jugular foramen |
| Vagus nerve (X) | Jugular foramen |
| Accessory nerve (XI) | Jugular foramen |
| Hypoglossal nerve (XII) | Hypoglossal foramen |

## CEREBELLUM

| | |
|---|---|
| **Name the two major functions of the cerebellum.** | Coordination and balance |
| **Localize each in the cerebellum.** | Coordination—cerebellar hemispheres<br>Balance—cerebellar vermis |
| **Do cerebellar lesions cause a sensory deficit?** | No. Clinically, it is only a motor structure. |
| **What is the cerebellum's arterial blood supply?** | Vertebrobasilar arterial system |

## BRAIN STEM

| | |
|---|---|
| **How is the brain stem similar to the spinal cord?** | It is the intracranial, upward extension of the cord. |
| **How does understanding the organization of the spinal cord help in understanding the brain stem?** | Brain stem organization is analogous to a complicated spinal cord. |
| **What are the three functional components in the spinal cord?** | Descending pathways, ascending pathways, and peripheral nerves |
| **Compare the four major functional components of the brain stem with the three major functional components of the spinal cord.** | The spinal cord and brain stem both have<br>    Descending motor pathways<br>    Ascending sensory pathways<br>    Peripheral nerves/cranial nerves<br>The brain stem also has the reticular formation. |

## THE SPINAL CORD IN THE VERTEBRAE

| | |
|---|---|
| **From top to bottom, what are the four divisions of the spinal cord?** | 1. Cervical cord<br>2. Thoracic cord<br>3. Lumbar cord<br>4. Sacral cord, which includes the conus medullaris |
| **What is the cauda equina?** | The "horse's tail" containing lumbar and sacral peripheral nerve roots that hangs below the tip of the spinal cord. |
| **At which vertebral body does the adult spinal cord end?** | About L1 |
| **What is the conus medullaris?** | The most inferior portion of the spinal cord |

## NEUROANATOMIC BASIS OF THE NEUROLOGIC EXAMINATION

## HIGHER COGNITIVE FUNCTION EXAMINATION

### The Cerebral Hemispheres

**What are higher cognitive functions?**

Brain functions that are integral for thinking

**At what level of the nervous system do lesions cause cognitive abnormalities?**

Cerebral cortex

**During which part of the neurologic examination are abnormalities of higher cognitive function assessed?**

Mental status examination

**What five cognitive functions are routinely examined in a neurologic mental status examination?**

Level of consciousness, orientation, memory, language, and praxis

**What is topographic localization?**

The assignment of a specific neurologic function to a specific anatomic site

**What is an example of topographic localization in the cerebral cortex?**

The cortex of the calcarine fissure in the occipital lobe is the visual receptive area.

**What is "primary" cortex?**

A region of cortex devoted to a *single* sensory or motor function, such as the occipital visual cortex

**What are six primary cortical functions?**

1. Movement (somatic motor cortex)
2. Sensation (somatosensory cortex)
3. Visual function
4. Auditory function
5. Gustatory function
6. Olfactory function

| | |
|---|---|
| **What is "secondary" cortex?** | A region of cortex devoted to more complex functions of a single sensory or motor modality. It is typically adjacent to the primary cortex for that modality. |
| **What is "association" cortex?** | A region of cortex devoted to integrating different sensory and motor modalities. It is typically situated between secondary cortices, so that it can access them easily. It is involved in functions such as learning, emotion, and spatial manipulation. |

## The Brain by Lobes

| | |
|---|---|
| **What lobe of the brain contains the primary and secondary motor cortex?** | The frontal lobe |
| **What frontal lobe gyrus contains the primary motor cortex, or motor strip?** | The precentral gyrus |
| **What neurologic deficit is caused by a lesion here?** | Upper motor neuron (UMN) weakness |
| **What lobe of the brain contains the primary somatosensory cortex?** | The parietal lobe |
| **What parietal gyrus contains the primary sensory cortex?** | The postcentral gyrus |
| **What neurologic deficit is caused by a lesion here?** | "Cortical" sensory deficits, such as agraphesthesia and astereognosis |
| **What spatial function is contained in the remainder of the parietal lobe, particularly the inferior parietal lobule?** | Attention to contralateral hemispace. It is significantly stronger in the right inferior parietal lobule than in the left. |
| **What neurologic deficit is caused by a lesion here?** | Neglect syndrome |

| | |
|---|---|
| **How are sensory and visual neglect syndromes best elicited?** | Extinction to double simultaneous stimulation |
| **How is extinction to double simultaneous stimulation elicited?** | Simultaneous presentation of stimuli to the right and left sides. For example, show one finger in the right visual field and two fingers in the left visual field. If the patient only sees one finger, then they "extinguish" on the left. |
| **What other behaviors may be part of the neglect syndrome?** | Hemispatial neglect (e.g., imperfect drawing of the left side of a figure), anosognosia, hemiakinesia |
| **What other function is also contained in the parietal lobe?** | Praxis |
| **What is praxis?** | The ability to carry out complicated, learned motor activities, such as using utensils (e.g., hairbrush, toothbrush) or putting on clothes |
| **What is apraxia?** | The inability to carry out motor activities despite intact strength and sensation. Apraxia may be subdivided into constructional and ideomotor apraxia. |
| **What is -*gnosis* and *agnosia*?** | -*gnosis* means awareness of something. Therefore, *agnosia* is lack of awareness or inability to sense something. |
| **What is astereognosis?** | The inability to discern a three-dimensional object by touch without looking at it (e.g., inability to recognize a coin by examining it with the fingers) |
| **Finger agnosia?** | The inability to recognize named fingers properly |
| **Anosognosia?** | An individual's lack of awareness of a deficit |
| **What brain lobe contains the primary visual cortex?** | The occipital lobe |

**What fissure runs through the middle of the primary visual cortex?**

The calcarine fissure

**What neurologic deficit is caused by a unilateral lesion?**

Contralateral hemianopia

**What is contained in the remainder of the occipital lobe?**

Secondary (visual association) cortex

**What neurologic deficit is caused by a bilateral lesion?**

Anton's syndrome (cortical blindness), pupillary light reflexes are preserved

**What is characteristic about Anton's syndrome?**

The patients deny they are blind

**Where is the primary auditory cortex?**

The temporal lobe, in Heschl's transverse gyrus

**What neurologic deficit is caused by a unilateral temporal lesion here?**

Usually none, because sound is received bilaterally

**What are the two main speech areas of the brain?**

Broca's and Wernicke's areas

**In which hemisphere are they located?**

The dominant hemisphere, which is the left hemisphere for 95% of the population

**Where in the dominant hemisphere is language function located?**

It is localized along the banks of the Sylvian fissure.

**What is the arterial blood supply to this area?**

The middle cerebral artery

**The figure on the following page is an external view of the left hemisphere. Label the location of the Sylvian fissure and Broca's and Wernicke's areas.**

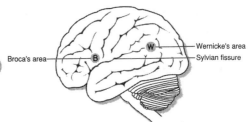

| | |
|---|---|
| **What is aphasia?** | A disturbance of language processing caused by CNS injury |
| **What aspects of language should be tested in a brief clinical examination for aphasia?** | Remember the mnemonic SCRAWL **S**pontaneous speech–fluency, effort, paraphasic errors **C**omprehension **R**epetition **A**nomia **W**riting **L**exical (reading) |
| **How is aphasia different from dysarthria?** | Dysarthria refers to impaired articulation of speech and does not imply an acquired defect of language |
| **Name the two most important aphasias.** | Broca's aphasia and Wernicke's fluent aphasia |
| **What do they have in common?** | Poor ability to repeat |
| **Characterize Broca's aphasia.** | Nonfluent aphasia (effortful, short phrase length, decreased rate), with impaired repetition but preserved comprehension |
| **Localize the usual lesion of Broca's aphasia.** | Inferior frontal lobe of dominant hemisphere |
| **Characterize Wernicke's aphasia.** | Fluent aphasia (normal rate), with impaired comprehension and repetition and marked paraphasias |
| **Localize the usual lesion of Wernicke's aphasia.** | Posterior superior temporal lobe of dominant hemisphere |
| **Name two other aphasias.** | Transcortical and conduction |

**Characterize transcortical aphasia.**

Aphasia with preserved ability to repeat

**Localize the usual lesion of transcortical aphasia.**

Adjacent to, but not including, Broca's or Wernicke's area.

**Characterize conduction aphasia.**

Aphasia with markedly impaired repetition, but preserved fluency and comprehension

**How does the ability to repeat help to localize language deficits?**

Impaired repetition implies perisylvian pathology. Preserved repetition in an aphasic patient suggests the injury is away from the Sylvian fissure (e.g., as occurs in watershed infarcts).

**Which aphasia is most common?**

Broca's nonfluent aphasia

**Review typical aphasic syndromes according to speech fluency and comprehension as well as the ability to repeat.**

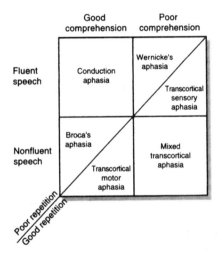

This figure will help you remember features of typical aphasic syndromes, but it should not be used to force individual aphasic patients into categories. A clinical description of a patient's language deficits (i.e., SCRAWL) is more useful.

**On the following figure, name the aphasia caused by a lesion in each numbered area.**

1. Broca's, nonfluent aphasia
2. Wernicke's fluent aphasia
3. Conduction aphasia
4. and 5. Transcortical aphasia

1. _____
2. _____
3. _____
4. _____
5. _____

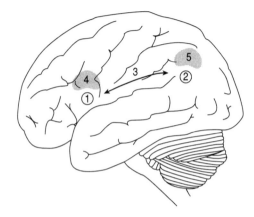

**What functions are represented in the prefrontal cortex?**

Control of emotion and social interactions

**What is an example of a disease that preferentially affects the frontal lobe?**

Pick's disease

**What are three frontal lobe release signs that may be present in patients with frontal lobe pathology (e.g., dementia)?**

Grasp, glabellar, and palmomental reflexes

## CRANIAL NERVE EXAMINATION

### Olfactory Nerve (CN I)

**What sensory function is mediated by the olfactory nerve?**

Smell

**How is it tested?**

By presenting strong odors to one nostril at a time. Commonly used stimuli include coffee, lemon, and clove.

| | |
|---|---|
| **When is olfactory testing indicated?** | If lesions of the olfactory nerve are suspected (e.g., following head injury that may have severed the olfactory nerve) |
| **Why isn't smell tested routinely?** | Disorders of CN I are uncommon; smell is commonly impaired by obstruction of nasal passages and is often lost in the elderly. |

## Visual Pathways and Pupillary Light Reflex (CN II)

| | |
|---|---|
| **How is visual acuity tested?** | By presenting appropriate stimuli to each eye. At bedside, the clinician asks the patient to read letters on a standardized hand-held card. |
| **When testing neurologic optic pathway function, should the patient wear his prescription glasses if he has them?** | Yes |
| **Why?** | Poor visual acuity caused by retinal or optic pathway dysfunction is not correctable by refraction. Poor visual acuity that is corrected with refraction through eyeglasses is usually caused by abnormalities in the lens or other parts of the refraction system. |
| **What is hemianopia?** | Visual field defect (or "cut") involving half of the visual field |
| **Are hemianopsia and hemianopia the same defect?** | Yes |
| **What is a homonymous hemianopia?** | Visual field cut involving the same half of the visual field in each eye |
| **In the pathway used for vision, where is the first synapse after the retina?** | Lateral geniculate body |

**Draw the visual field seen by each eye of a patient with a right homonymous hemianopsia.**

Left eye 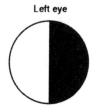     Right eye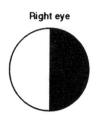

**Where in the visual pathway would there be a lesion that causes monocular blindness?**

Ipsilateral eye or optic nerve before it reaches the chiasm ("prechiasmatic")

**Where in the visual pathway would there be a lesion that causes bitemporal hemianopsia?**

At the optic chiasm (e.g., a pituitary tumor)

**Where in the visual pathway would there be a lesion that causes right superior quadrantanopsia?**

Left (contralateral) inferior bank of the calcarine cortex

**Where in the visual pathway would there be a lesion that causes right homonymous hemianopsia?**

Left (contralateral) hemisphere, both inferior and superior

**What is optokinetic nystagmus?**

Nystagmus produced by moving a vertically striped stimulus horizontally across the visual field

**Describe the normal response.**

Nystagmus with the fast phase opposite to the direction of the stimulus, because the eyes track the stimulus across the visual field and then quickly saccade back to pick up and follow the stimulus again

**Can a malingering person suppress optokinetic nystagmus?**

Only with poor fixation

**How is pupillary light reflex tested?**

By shining a light in the eye and examining the ipsilateral and contralateral pupil

| | |
|---|---|
| **What is the term for unequal pupil size?** | Anisocoria |
| **Which parts of the autonomic nervous system mediate pupil size?** | The sympathetic and parasympathetic |
| **What is the function of the sympathetic innervation versus parasympathetic innervation?** | Sympathetic–pupillodilation<br>Parasympathetic–pupilloconstriction |
| **Where do the parasympathetic fibers in CN III originate?** | Near the CN III nucleus in the midbrain (Edinger-Westphal) |
| **How do the parasympathetic fibers reach the eye?** | They travel with the oculomotor nerve (CN III). |
| **What pupil abnormality is caused by dysfunction or disease of the parasympathetic innervation to the pupil?** | Ipsilateral large unreactive pupil (mydriasis) |
| **Where in the brain do the sympathetic fibers originate?** | Hypothalamus |
| **Trace the sympathetic pathway from the brain to the spinal cord.** | From the hypothalamus, it descends through lateral brain stem and lateral spinal cord. |
| **Where in the spinal cord do the sympathetic paths synapse before exiting?** | Intermediolateral cell column of low cervical and high thoracic cord |
| **Why is this structure called the intermediolateral cell column of grey matter?** | It is midway between the dorsal and ventral horns of the spinal cord, on the lateral (rather than medial) aspect of the grey matter. |
| **Where do sympathetic fibers go after leaving the spinal cord?** | To the "sympathetic chain" of ganglia in the paravertebral region of low cervical and high thoracic cord |
| **What is the most cephalad paravertebral ganglion?** | Superior cervical ganglion |

**Why is it especially important?**

It provides sympathetic fibers that eventually reach the pupillodilator muscle of the eye.

**How do the fibers get from the superior cervical ganglion to the eye?**

They ascend with the carotid artery back into the skull and then branch to the eye.

**What pupil abnormality is caused by dysfunction or disease of the sympathetic innervation to the pupil?**

Ipsilateral small pupil (miosis)

**In the pupillary light reflex pathway, where is the first synapse after the retina?**

Pretectal area of the brain stem

**Why does shining a light in only one eye cause both pupils to constrict?**

Fibers from each pretectal nucleus innervate the parasympathetic portions of both third cranial nerve nuclei, causing bilateral pupilloconstriction.

**Does unilateral retinal disease cause anisocoria?**

No, because the pretectal nucleus responds to whichever eye "sees" the greater amount of light

**What are the two prechiasmatic components of the visual system?**

Retina and optic nerve

**What test of pupillary light response is used to detect prechiasmatic dysfunction?**

The swinging flashlight test

**What is the normal response to this test?**

Shining a light in one eye causes ipsilateral and consensual pupillary constriction. Swinging the light to the other eye causes the same degree of constriction in the ipsilateral and consensual pupils.

**What is an abnormal response to this test?**

Shining a light in the affected eye causes a small amount of constriction in both the ipsilateral and consensual pupils. Swinging the light from the affected eye to the unaffected eye causes an increase in pupillary constriction of both pupils, because the pretectal nucleus now "sees" more light coming through the unaffected retina.

| What is this defect called? | Relative Afferent Pupillary Defect, or RAPD |
|---|---|

### Eye Movement (CN III, IV, and VI)

| Which cranial nerves innervate the extraocular muscles? | CN III, IV, and VI |
|---|---|

**Which extraocular muscles are innervated by each of these cranial nerves:**

| CN III? | Superior rectus, inferior rectus, medial rectus, inferior oblique |
|---|---|
| CN IV? | Superior oblique |
| CN VI? | Lateral rectus |
| What extraocular eye muscle (EOM) movement abnormality is caused by paresis of CN VI? | Unilateral inability to abduct the eye (i.e., inability to look laterally) |
| What EOM abnormality is caused by paresis of CN IV? | Unilateral inability to gaze downward, especially when the eye is adducted |
| What EOM abnormality is caused by paresis of CN III? | Unilateral inability to gaze upward or adduct the eye. Eye is "down and out." |
| What are two additional eye findings typically present with a complete third-nerve palsy? | 1. Dilated pupil caused by parasympathetic denervation<br>2. Ptosis caused by denervation of the levator palpebrae |
| In simplistic terms, what are the functions of CNs III, IV, and VI? | CN VI abducts the eye; CN IV moves the eye down and in; and CN III does everything else plus constricts the pupil and elevates the upper lid. |

On the following figure, fill in the blank with the name of the eye muscle and cranial nerve responsible for each primary direction of gaze.

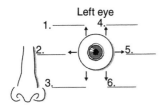

Left eye

1. Inferior oblique CN III
2. Medial rectus CN III
3. Superior oblique CN IV
4. Superior rectus CN III
5. Lateral rectus CN VI
6. Inferior rectus CN III

| | |
|---|---|
| **What anatomic region controls conjugate vertical gaze?** | Gaze center in the roof (tectum) of the midbrain |
| **What eye movement abnormality is caused by lesions of this region?** | Bilateral inability to look upward |
| **What is the eponym for impaired vertical gaze and pupillary light reflex that are caused by a lesion of the midbrain tectum?** | Parinaud's syndrome |
| **What gaze center is located in the frontal cortex?** | Horizontal gaze center in the frontal eye fields |
| **What aspect of horizontal gaze does it control?** | It "pushes" the eyes toward the contralateral direction |
| **What gaze abnormality is caused by a lesion of this area?** | Impaired conjugate gaze away from the side of the lesion, with consequent deviation of the eyes toward the side of the lesion |
| **To which direction will the eyes deviate in a left frontal stroke?** | To the left |

**What gaze center is in the pons?**

Pontine lateral gaze center; it is also called the pontine paramedian reticular formation (PPRF), or the para-abducens nucleus

**Where in the pons is it located?**

Adjacent to the CN VI nucleus

**What aspect of horizontal gaze does it control?**

It pulls the eyes in the ipsilateral direction

**What gaze abnormality is caused by a lesion of this area?**

Impaired conjugate gaze toward the side of the lesion, with consequent deviation away from the side of the lesion

**To which direction will the eyes deviate in a left brain stem stroke?**

To the right if it involves the left lateral gaze center

**To which direction do the eyes deviate in a frontal stroke versus a brain stem stroke?**

In a frontal stroke, the eyes *look at* the lesion; in a brain stem stroke, the eyes *look away from* the lesion.

**What muscles and cranial nerves are used in gazing toward the left?**

Left CN VI controls the lateral rectus of the left eye. Right CN III controls the medial rectus of the right eye.

**Through which pathway are they connected to permit coordinated lateral gaze?**

Medial longitudinal fasciculus (MLF)

**Where do the axons of the MLF originate?**

Pontine lateral gaze center

**Where do they cross the midline?**

In the pons, soon after leaving the pontine lateral gaze center

**What gaze abnormality is caused by a lesion of the right MLF?**

Inability to adduct the right (ipsilateral) eye past the midline, caused by the inability of the left CN VI nucleus to communicate with the right CN III nucleus

**What is the name for this neurologic sign?**

Internuclear ophthalmoplegia (INO)

On the following figure, draw the pathway between the frontal gaze center and the CN III and VI nuclei.

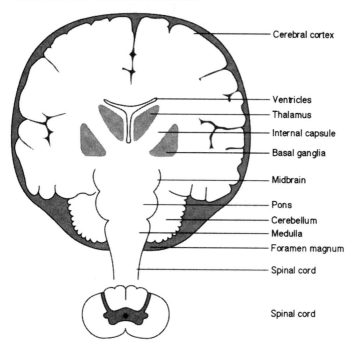

Cerebral cortex

Ventricles
Thalamus
Internal capsule
Basal ganglia

Midbrain

Pons
Cerebellum
Medulla
Foramen magnum

Spinal cord

Spinal cord

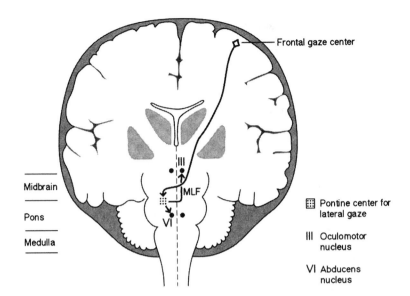

Frontal gaze center

Midbrain

Pons

Medulla

III MLF

VI

⊞ Pontine center for lateral gaze

III Oculomotor nucleus

VI Abducens nucleus

## Trigeminal Nerve (CN V)

**What is the sensory distribution of CN V?**

The face

**What are the three subdivisions of CN V, and what are their sensory distributions?**

1. Ophthalmic ($V_1$)–forehead and periorbital region
2. Maxillary ($V_2$)–central face around the nose
3. Mandibular ($V_3$)–jaw

**What is another name for trigeminal neuralgia?**

Tic douloureux

**What is it?**

Acute, brief lancinating pains in the trigeminal distribution, typically $V_2$

**What muscles are innervated by CN V, and how are they tested?**

**Pterygoid muscles** move the jaw laterally and are tested when the patient pushes the jaw laterally against the examiner's hand. **Masseter** and **temporalis muscles** close the jaw and are tested when the examiner pushes the jaw open against a closed mouth.

## Facial Nerve (CN VII)

**What does the facial nerve supply?**

Muscles of facial expression

**How are they tested?**

The patient is asked to wrinkle his forehead (or look upward), close his eyes, wrinkle his nose, and purse his lips.

**What neurologic deficit is caused by a lesion of the CN VII nucleus?**

Weakness of the ipsilateral upper and lower face; LMN weakness

**What neurologic deficit is caused by a lesion of CN VII after it leaves the brain stem?**

Weakness of the ipsilateral upper and lower face; LMN weakness

**What neurologic deficit is caused by a lesion of the corticobulbar fibers above the CN VII nucleus–i.e., a central VII lesion?**

Weakness of the lower half of face, sparing the upper half

| | |
|---|---|
| **Why?** | CN VII neurons that give rise to the fibers going to the upper half of the face receive bilateral corticobulbar UMN input. Thus, a unilateral UMN lesion does not completely denervate them. |
| **Name a special sensory function carried with CN VII.** | Taste |
| **From what part of the tongue?** | The anterior two thirds |

## Vestibulocochlear Nerve (CN VIII)

| | |
|---|---|
| **What are the two special sensory functions of this nerve?** | Auditory and labyrinthine |
| **What is the purpose of the Weber tuning fork test?** | To determine if lateralized (i.e., asymmetric) hearing loss is present |
| **How is the Weber test performed?** | A vibrating tuning fork is placed at the center of the forehead, and the patient reports whether the sound appears to originate from the right, the left, or the center of the head. |
| **What is an abnormal response to this test?** | Lateralization of the sound to either side |
| **What does an abnormal response indicate?** | Sensorineural hearing loss (e.g., disease of acoustic nerve) or conductive hearing loss (e.g., disease of middle ear ossicles). Sound lateralizes away from the side of sensorineural hearing loss, because that acoustic nerve is not capable of "hearing" as well. The sound lateralizes toward the side of conductive hearing loss, because the auditory apparatus responds to bone conduction with less competition from ambient sounds, which are masked on that side. |

## Glossopharyngeal Nerve (CN IX)

| | |
|---|---|
| **What special sensory function does CN IX carry?** | Taste for the posterior one third of the tongue |

| | |
|---|---|
| **What is the purpose of the Rinne test?** | To examine air and bone sound conduction |
| **How is it performed?** | Place tuning fork on mastoid; when sound stops, move beside ear |
| **What response is normal?** | Air conduction is louder than bone |
| **What does an abnormal response indicate?** | Conductive hearing loss (ossicle disease) |
| **What somatic sensory function does CN IX carry?** | Sensation from the oropharynx |
| **What motor functions does CN IX serve?** | Innervation of some muscles of swallowing |
| **How are these motor functions tested?** | Symmetric elevation of the palate when the patient says "Ah"; presence of a gag response when touching the posterior oropharynx |

### Vagus Nerve (CN X)

| | |
|---|---|
| **What are two voluntary muscle groups innervated by CN X?** | 1. Swallowing muscles of the oropharynx<br>2. Vocal cord muscles via the recurrent laryngeal nerve |
| **How is this tested?** | 1. Symmetric elevation of the palate in response to a gag and in response to saying "Ah"; these are mixed CN IX and X functions<br>2. A falsetto "E" requires bringing the vocal cords together. This is a CN X (recurrent laryngeal branch) function. |
| **Which way does the palate elevate in a unilateral lesion of CN IX and X?** | Away from the side that has the damaged nerve; the affected side does not elevate |
| **Which way does the uvula deviate in a unilateral lesion of CNs IX and X?** | Away from the side that has the damaged nerve; it is pulled toward the unaffected side |
| **What is an important autonomic function carried by CN X?** | Parasympathetic fibers are carried to most of the abdominal organs |

## Spinal Accessory Nerve (CN XI)

**What motor function is supplied by CN XI?**

Somatic motor fibers are supplied to the trapezius and sternocleidomastoid muscles

**How does a lesion of CN XI manifest on physical examination?**

The patient has weakness when shrugging her shoulders and turning her head

**To which direction does the head turn when the right sternocleidomastoid muscle is activated?**

To the left. You can remember this by putting your right thumb on your right sternum and your right index finger on your right mastoid process. When you pull them together with your right hand, your head turns to the left.

## Hypoglossal Nerve (CN XII)

**What is the function of CN XII?**

It carries motor fibers to the muscles of the tongue.

**Where is the nucleus of CN XII?**

In the paramedian medulla oblongata

**What is unique about the location of this cranial nerve nucleus compared with the others?**

It is the only somatic motor nucleus primarily in the medulla.

**How does a lesion of CN XII manifest?**

Deviation of the tongue toward the weak side

**Why?**

Tongue muscles act as if to "push" the tongue out, so the strong half of the tongue overcomes the weak half and deviates the tongue toward the weak side.

## MOTOR SYSTEM EXAMINATION

On the following figure of a coronal section of brain through motor cortex, label the motor homunculus for the sites of the UMN cell bodies to the leg, trunk, hand, face, lips, and pharynx.

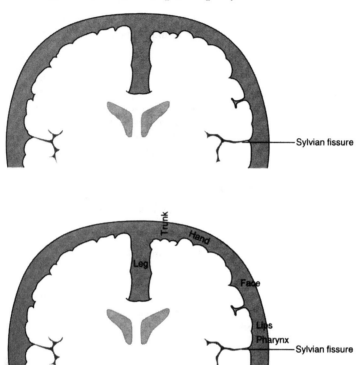

In the external and coronal view of the left hemisphere, name the body area served by the upper motor neurons in each numbered site.

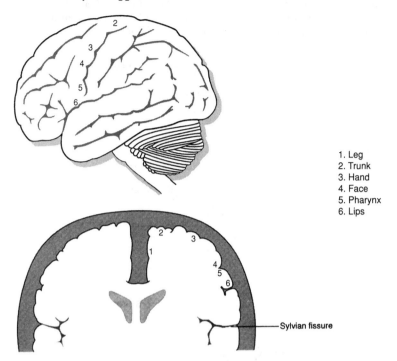

1. Leg
2. Trunk
3. Hand
4. Face
5. Pharynx
6. Lips

Sylvian fissure

On the following figure, draw the upper and lower motor paths as they pass from the cerebral motor cortex through subcortical white matter, internal capsule, pons, and medulla, to the spinal cord, and then out to a muscle. Identify the UMN and the LMN and the location of their cell bodies. Carefully specify where they cross the midline.

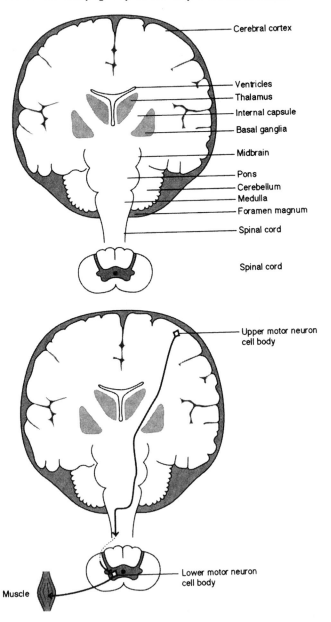

| | |
|---|---|
| **Where does the UMN path cross the midline?** | Primarily in the pyramidal decussation of the low medulla |
| **Where is this area in relation to the skull?** | Immediately above the foramen magnum |
| **Where is the first synapse in the direct corticospinal path?** | Anterior horn of spinal cord |

**What is the main spinal cord level that contributes motor nerve fibers to each of the following muscles of the upper extremity:**

| | |
|---|---|
| Deltoid? | C5 |
| Biceps? | C5–C6 |
| Triceps? | C7 |
| Interossei (intrinsic hand muscles)? | C8–T1 |

| | |
|---|---|
| **What is the action of each of these muscles?** | The deltoid abducts the shoulder; the biceps flexes the elbow; the triceps extends the elbow; and the interossei abduct and adduct outstretched fingers. |
| **How are these muscles tested?** | 1. Deltoid: push down on the patient's arms, which are outstretched at 90° <br> 2. Biceps: pull on the patient's forearm with the elbow flexed at 90° <br> 3. Triceps: push against the patient's forearm with the elbow flexed at 90° <br> 4. Interossei: push the patient's fingers together when they are abducted fully |
| **What spinal cord levels and nerve roots are tested by the biceps reflex?** | C5, C6 |
| **The brachioradialis reflex?** | C5, C6 |
| **The triceps reflex?** | C7 |

| | |
|---|---|
| **What spatial characteristic does this sequence of muscles have?** | They are arranged sequentially from proximal to distal in the arm and involve each joint progressively down the arm, correlating with progressively more inferior spinal cord levels. |

**What is the main spinal cord level that contributes motor nerve fibers to each of the following muscles?**

| | |
|---|---|
| **Iliopsoas?** | L1 |
| **Leg adductors?** | L2 |
| **Quadriceps?** | L3–L4 |
| **Tibialis anterior?** | L4–L5 |
| **Tibialis posterior?** | L5 |
| **Gastrocnemius?** | S1 |

| | |
|---|---|
| **What is the action of each of these muscles?** | The iliopsoas flexes the hip; the leg adductors bring the knees together; the quadriceps extends the knee; the tibialis anterior dorsiflexes the foot; the tibialis posterior everts the foot; and the gastrocnemius plantar-flexes the foot. |

| | |
|---|---|
| **What spinal cord levels and nerve roots are tested by the patellar (knee jerk) reflex?** | L3, L4 |
| **The Achilles (ankle jerk) reflex?** | S1 |
| **What spatial characteristic does this sequence of muscles have?** | They are arranged sequentially from proximal to distal in the leg and involve each joint progressively down the leg. |
| **Why is this sequence important to know?** | It helps localize the level of a spinal cord lesion. Moving from proximal to distal helps remind you which spinal segment innervates which muscles. |

**Describe the circuit traversed by the impulse that is initiated when testing the deep tendon reflex.**

A tap on the tendon quickly stretches the muscle activating the muscle spindles. They project back to and activate the anterior horn cells of spinal cord. These motor neurons fire a signal down to the muscle, causing it to contract.

**Where do you localize an injury of the UMN?**

Anywhere above the anterior horn cell

**What are four common UMN signs?**

Spasticity, hyperreflexia, Babinski's sign, and weakness

**Where do you localize an injury of the LMN?**

At or below the anterior horn cell

**What are five common LMN signs?**

Hypotonia, hyporeflexia, atrophy, fasciculations, and weakness

**What are the motor signs of a focal lesion of the spinal cord?**

LMN signs in muscles innervated by injured anterior horn cells and UMN signs in muscles innervated below the injured segment

**Why do UMN signs occur below the injured segment of the spinal cord?**

The corticospinal tract is injured on its way down through the lesion, but the anterior horn cells to which it is going are intact below the lesion.

**What is the utility of the jaw jerk reflex?**

The reflex is tested by tapping on the patient's jaw while he holds it half open. Hyperactivity indicates UMN lesion above the pons.

**What is the utility of abdominal reflexes?**

These reflexes are tested by briskly stroking the skin of the abdomen. Absence of these reflexes indicates UMN disease above the thoracic spinal cord.

**What is the utility of the bulbocavernosus reflex?**

This reflex is tested when the examiner squeezes the patient's glans penis and feels the anal sphincter contract against his finger. Absence of this reflex indicates sacral cord disease.

## SENSORY SYSTEM EXAMINATION

| | |
|---|---|
| **Where is the primary sensory cortex?** | Postcentral gyrus of the parietal lobe |
| **What are the two main ascending long tracts of the spinal cord that carry sensation?** | The dorsal columns and spinothalamic tracts receive peripheral sensory input |
| **Where do both tracts synapse before ascending up to the parietal lobe cortex?** | Thalamus |
| **Where are the bipolar neurons that give rise to both tracts?** | Paravertebral dorsal root ganglia |
| **Which tract then has its next synapse close to level of entry?** | Spinothalamic |
| **Which tract then has its next synapse at the level of foramen magnum?** | Dorsal columns |
| **What then is the course of both tracts?** | Decussate and ascend to cortex via thalamus |
| **Which three primary sensory modalities are carried by the dorsal column pathway?** | Vibration, proprioception, and gross touch |
| **Which three primary sensory modalities are carried by the spinothalmic pathways?** | Pain, temperature, and light touch |

On the following figure, draw the sensory fibers of the *dorsal column* pathway from the sensory receptors in the fingers up to the primary sensory cortex. Include in your drawing each of the following components: sensory organ, peripheral sensory nerve, dorsal root ganglion, dorsal horn of spinal cord, dorsal column in spinal cord (cuneate), cuneate nucleus, decussation of dorsal columns, thalamus, and the primary sensory cortex. There are four nerve cell bodies in this pathway. Carefully specify where the pathway crosses the midline.

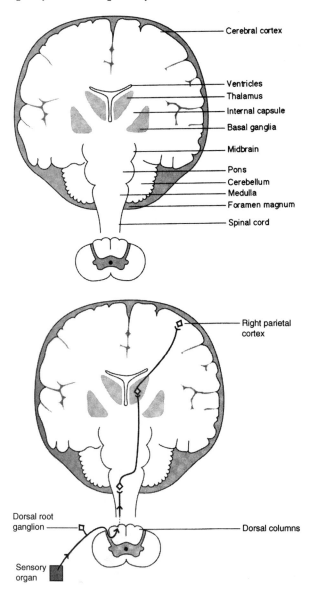

Cerebral cortex

Ventricles
Thalamus
Internal capsule
Basal ganglia

Midbrain

Pons
Cerebellum
Medulla
Foramen magnum

Spinal cord

Right parietal cortex

Dorsal root ganglion

Dorsal columns

Sensory organ

**At what level does the dorsal column decussate?**

Cervicomedullary junction

**What are the Latin names for each of the two dorsal columns.**

Cuneatus and gracilis

**How do you remember which dorsal column carries upper extremity sensation and which carries lower extremity sensation?**

CCC—The cuneatus carries cervical fibers from the upper extremity. They enter the cord above those of the lower extremity and are lateral in the cord.

**On which nucleus of the thalamus do axons from sensory paths synapse?**

Ventral posterior nucleus. It is divided into ventral posterior lateral (VPL) and ventral posterior medial (VPM) nuclei. VP**L** serves the body, and VPM serves the face. The body is **L**ower than the face.

**How can you remember the location of the upper body dermatomes?**

Eight upper body dermatomes correspond with easily identifiable anatomic landmarks:
C1–doesn't exist
C2–back of head
C4–above collar bone
C6–thumb
C7–middle fingers
C8–little finger
T4–nipple line
T10–umbilicus

**How can you remember the location of the lower body dermatomes?**

Remember the *dermatome dance.* Put your hands over L1 and move to successive dermatomes, which more or less circumnavigate the leg:
L1–groin
L2–lateral thigh
L3–medial thigh
L4–medial leg
L5–lateral leg, big toe
S1–little toe, sole of foot

**What is the term for the pattern of innervation of a muscle by a spinal nerve root?**

Radicular distribution; it is equivalent to dermatomal sensory distributions

**What are the three most important peripheral nerves in the upper extremity that are both sensory and motor?**

Radial, median, ulnar

**What are the two most important peripheral nerves in the leg that are both sensory and motor?**

Femoral, peroneal

On the following figure, draw the sensory fibers from the sensory organs in the skin up the *spinothalamic tract* of the spinal cord, to the primary sensory cortex. Include in your drawing each of the following components: sensory receptors in the fingers, peripheral sensory nerve, dorsal root ganglion, dorsal horn of spinal cord, decussation in the ventral white matter of spinal cord, lateral spinothalamic tract, thalamus, and the primary sensory cortex. There are four cell bodies in this pathway.

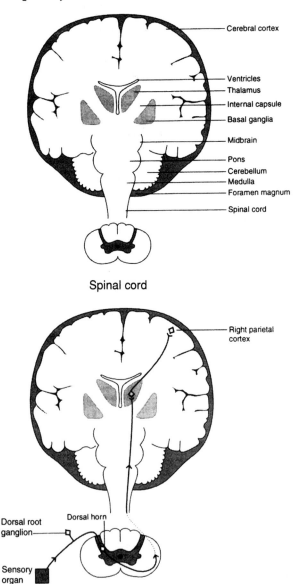

**Using the figure below on the left, label the following sensory dermatomes: C2, C4, C6, C7, C8, T4, T10, L1, L2, L3, L4, L5, S1, and S5.**

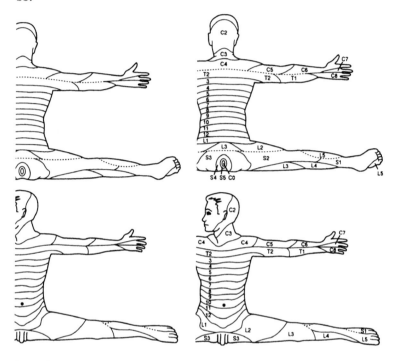

(Reproduced and adapted with permission from Haymaker W, Woodhall B: *Peripheral Nerve Injuries.* 2nd ed. Philadelphia, WB Saunders, 1953, p 19.)

On the following figure, identify the cutaneous sensory distribution of these five peripheral nerves: (1) radial, (2) median, (3) ulnar, (4) femoral, and (5) peroneal.

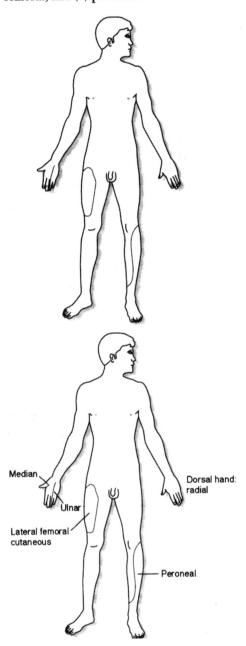

## COORDINATION EXAMINATION

| | |
|---|---|
| **What is the most important part of the brain that contributes to coordination?** | Cerebellum |
| **What other four systems must be intact before attributing incoordination to cerebellar dysfunction?** | 1. Vision: it provides clues to help coordinate movement<br>2. Motor system: strength must be sufficient to perform the specified task<br>3. Sensation (especially proprioception): the patient must be able to detect where the limbs are<br>4. Vestibular system: the patient must be able to integrate rotational movement and neck muscles |
| **What part of the cerebellum is most important for control of leg coordination?** | Vermis |
| **What parts of the cerebellum are most important for arm and hand coordination?** | The hemispheres |
| **What are four signs that suggest cerebellar incoordination?** | Dysmetria, intention tremor, ataxia, dysdiadochokinesis (impaired rapid alternating movements) |
| **What is dysmetria?** | Incoordination that manifests as jerky, arrhythmic irregular movement when the affected individual tries to perform a task or reach a target |
| **How is it elicited in the upper extremities?** | By asking the patient to alternately touch his nose and then the examiner's fingers, which are placed at arm's length |
| **How is dysmetria different from intention tremor?** | Intention tremor is a fine rhythmic, regular movement of the outstretched finger that intensifies as the patient tries to touch the examiner's finger. |

**How is ataxia elicited?**

By observing the patient walking; it may be precipitated by walking with one foot in front of the other, "as though walking on a line," or "the drunk test"

## Lateral Medullary Infarction or Wallenberg's Syndrome

A very complex stroke syndrome, it consists of brain stem and cerebellar manifestations, without arm or leg paralysis or altered consciousness. It is located in the lower brain stem and due to ischemia of the lateral medulla which is nourished by the posterior inferior cerebellar artery. It originates from the vertebral.

The many signs and symptoms result from infarction of nuclei and tracts which, however, spare CN XII and the corticospinal tracts.

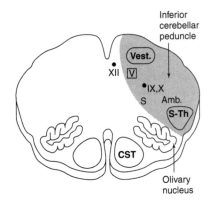

*CST*: corticospinal tract in pyramid; *Amb*: nucleus ambiguus (IX and X);
S: descending sympathetic pathway from hypothalamus to T-1; *vest*: vestibular nucleus
V: descending (spinal) nucleus C.N.V.; *S-Th*: ascending lateral spinothalamic tract.

# 4

# Differential Diagnosis of Common Problems

## HEADACHE

**What is the important difference between functional and symptomatic headache?**

Functional—no discernable structural disease

Symptomatic (or organic)—structural disease is present

**Name three common functional headaches.**

1. Tension or muscle contraction headache
2. Vascular headache, including migraine and cluster
3. Chronic daily headache

**Name four important causes of symptomatic headaches.**

1. Increased intracranial pressure
2. Intracerebral hemorrhage
3. Subarachnoid hemorrhage
4. CNS infection

**Which is more common, functional or symptomatic headache?**

95% of headache patients have functional headache

**What are two features that suggest a serious cause of headache?**

Abnormal neurologic examination and recent onset

**What are three important causes of elevated intracranial pressure?**

Mass lesion (e.g., tumor), pseudotumor cerebri, hydrocephalus

**At what time of day is a brain tumor headache often most severe?**

On first awakening

**What eye sign best identifies elevated intracranial pressure in a patient with headaches?**

Papilledema

**What disease may cause headache with papilledema when no mass lesion is present?**

Pseudotumor cerebri (also called benign intracranial hypertension)

**What distinguishes a complicated migraine from other migraines?**

A complicated migraine has focal neurologic signs, such as hemiparesis.

**What distinguishes a classic from a common migraine?**

A visual aura accompanies or precedes classic migraine.

**What clinical feature distinguishes cluster headaches from other headaches?**

Frequent severe nocturnal pain, often associated with facial autonomic symptoms

**Name three facial pain syndromes.**

Trigeminal neuralgia, temporal (giant cell) arteritis, temporomandibular joint (TMJ) pain

**What distinguishes facial pain syndromes from headache syndromes?**

Pain is primarily in the face, not the cranium.

**What is a serious cause of unilateral head pain accompanied by elevated ESR?**

Temporal arteritis (also called giant cell arteritis or cranial arteritis)

**Localize the pain of temporal arteritis.**

Just above the ear piece of eyeglasses

**Why is temporal arteritis an important diagnosis to consider?**

May cause blindness from ophthalmic artery involvement if not treated promptly

**What is the most common cause of lancinating facial pain?**

Trigeminal neuralgia

**What character of the pain distinguishes TMJ pain from other face pains?**

Pain and tenderness in the TMJ

| What relieves post–dural puncture headache ( "LP headache")? | Lying down—also see L.P. headache pages 109 and 259 |
|---|---|

**Table 4–1.   Do-It-Yourself Differential Diagnosis of Headache**

| Symptomatic | Elevated ICP: mass lesion, pseudotumor, hydrocephalus<br>Hemorrhage: intracerebral, subarachnoid<br>CNS infection |
|---|---|
| Functional | Vascular headache: migraine (classic, common, complicated), cluster<br>Tension (muscle contraction) headache<br>Chronic daily headache |
| Facial pain syndromes | Trigeminal neuralgia<br>Temporal arteritis<br>Temporomandibular joint (TMJ) pain |

## DEMENTIA

| What are four causes of insidious onset (chronic) dementia? | Alzheimer's disease, multi-infarct dementia, vitamin $B_{12}$ deficiency, neurosyphilis |
|---|---|
| Are there clinical characteristics that specifically identify Alzheimer's disease? | No. It is a diagnosis of exclusion. |
| What clinical characteristic usually distinguishes multi-infarct dementia? | Step-wise progression of symptoms |
| What clinical characteristics usually distinguish vitamin $B_{12}$ deficiency? | Associated sensory symptoms caused by peripheral neuropathy, or subacute degeneration of spinal cord, or RBC macrocytosis |
| What clinical characteristics usually distinguish neurosyphilis? | Associated sensory symptoms caused by tabes dorsalis and a positive blood or CSF test for syphilis |
| What are three causes of subacute onset of dementia? | Normal pressure hydrocephalus, Creutzfeldt-Jakob disease, Lewy body dementia |

**What clinical characteristics distinguish Creutzfeldt-Jakob disease?**

Associated myoclonus and periodic discharges on EEG in an adult

**What clinical characteristics usually distinguish normal pressure hydrocephalus?**

Associated gait ataxia and incontinence

**What are two inherited causes of dementia and movement disorder?**

Huntington's disease, Wilson's disease

**Table 4–2.   Do-It-Yourself Differential Diagnosis of Dementia**

| Symptom Duration | Disease | Associated Findings |
| --- | --- | --- |
| Chronic | Alzheimer's disease | None |
| | Multi-infarct dementia | Step-wise progression often |
| | Vitamin $B_{12}$ deficiency | Low vitamin $B_{12}$, macrocytosis, sensory symptoms |
| | Neurosyphilis | Positive tests for syphilis |
| Subacute | Normal-pressure hydrocephalus | Ataxia, incontinence |
| | Creutzfeldt-Jacob disease | Myoclonus, periodic EEG discharges |
| | Lewy body dementia | Visual hallucinations |
| Dementia and Movement Disorder | Huntington's disease | Positive family history and genetic tests |
| | Wilson's disease | Low ceruloplasmin, Kayser-Fleischer rings |

## ALTERED MENTAL STATUS

**Define altered mental status.**

Acute encephalopathy; any change in alertness or cognition, ranging from confusion to coma

**List five common neurologic disorders that cause altered mental status.**

1. Metabolic encephalopathy
2. Seizures
3. Stroke
4. Anoxic encephalopathy
5. Infection

**Which of these is the most common cause of mild persistent confusion?**

Metabolic encephalopathy

## METABOLIC ENCEPHALOPATHY

| | |
|---|---|
| **Define metabolic encephalopathy.** | Brain dysfunction of metabolic or toxic cause, usually without focal neurologic deficits |
| **What is the most common cause of metabolic encephalopathy in hospitalized patients?** | Drugs |
| **What are three other general medical causes of metabolic encephalopathy?** | 1. Infection (e.g., CNS or systemic infection)<br>2. Organ failure (e.g., hepatic or renal failure)<br>3. Deficiency states (e.g., Wernicke's encephalopathy, hypoglycemia, hyperglycemia) |
| **List two causes of altered mental status in fulminant hepatic failure.** | 1. Cerebral edema with increased ICP (also in Reye's syndrome)<br>2. Excess ammonia |
| **What is the most common movement disorder associated with chronic hepatic failure?** | Asterixis |
| **What is asterixis?** | Momentary loss of muscle tone ("flapping") |
| **What does it look like?** | With arms and wrists extended, the patient's hands briefly flap downward |
| **What causes lethargy in renal failure?** | Elevated BUN (uremia) |
| **What is the dialysis disequilibrium syndrome?** | Headache, confusion, somnolence; usually with large fluid/solute shifts |
| **What signs, in addition to confusion, suggest Wernicke's encephalopathy?** | Abnormalities of eye movements (e.g., nystagmus, ophthalmoplegia) and ataxia |
| **How is it diagnosed and treated?** | Improvement of signs in response to thiamine strongly supports the diagnosis |

**What eight laboratory tests are most useful in evaluating altered mental status in hospitalized patients?**

Glucose, CBC, liver enzyme tests, electrolytes, BUN, arterial blood gas, serum drug levels, lumbar puncture for CSF

**What test result abnormalities would help explain an altered mental state?**

Glucose—hypoglycemia, nonketotic hyperglycemia
CBC—leukocytosis (infection), anemia
Liver enzyme tests—elevated transaminases (hepatitis, liver failure)
Electrolytes—hyponatremia
BUN—uremia
ABG—hypoxia
Serum drug levels—antiepileptic, digoxin, or other specific drug toxicity
CSF—increased WBCs, increased protein, decreased glucose (infection)

## SEIZURES

**What is the term for confusion or lethargy following a seizure?**

Postictal state

**What is its characteristic time course?**

Usually brief, ranging from a few minutes to 1 hour, although prolonged postictal states rarely occur

**What rare type of seizure causes a persistently altered mental state without obvious motor seizures?**

Nonconvulsive status epilepticus

**How is it diagnosed?**

EEG demonstrates seizure discharges while the patient is confused. Also, both the confusion and EEG discharges resolve with intravenous diazepam.

## STROKE

**How is confusion caused by stroke distinguished from that caused by metabolic encephalopathy?**

Stroke is usually associated with focal neurologic signs.

| | |
|---|---|
| **What is the mechanism of impaired consciousness in stroke?** | Edema at the site of infarction causes mass effect. The edema causes pressure either on the other hemisphere, resulting in bihemispheric dysfunction, or on the brain stem's reticular activating system (RAS). |
| **Name two focal brain lesions whose clinical manifestations may be confused with altered mental status.** | 1. Aphasia (dominant hemisphere lesion) 2. Neglect (non-dominant parietal lesion) |
| **Which two causes of metabolic encephalopathy may cause *focal* neurologic signs or partial seizures and thus mimic stroke?** | Hypoglycemia; nonketotic hyperglycemia |
| **Who is at highest risk of developing a chronic subdural hematoma (SDH)?** | The elderly |
| **Why can it cause confusion without obvious focal findings?** | Its slow onset may permit the brain to shift and avoid localized pressure |
| **How is stroke best distinguished from SDH?** | By head CT or MRI |

## ANOXIC ENCEPHALOPATHY

| | |
|---|---|
| **What is the most common cause of anoxic encephalopathy?** | Cardiac arrest |
| **What is post–anoxic encephalopathy?** | Persistently altered mental state originally caused by brain anoxia |
| **How is post–anoxic encephalopathy distinguished from other encephalopathies?** | History of an anoxic insult |
| **What motor movement often accompanies post–anoxic encephalopathy?** | Myoclonus |

| | |
|---|---|
| **Generally, what is the prognosis for functional recovery?** | Poor |
| **How is ongoing hypoxia diagnosed?** | Low oxygen saturation by a pulse oximeter or low $P_{O_2}$ on ABG |

**Table 4–3.**
**Do-It-Yourself Differential Diagnosis of Altered Mental Status**

| Etiology | Comments |
|---|---|
| Metabolic encephalopathy | |
|   Drugs | Benzodiazepines, barbiturates, narcotics |
|   Toxins | Ethyl alcohol, drugs of abuse |
|   Organ failure | Hepatic, renal |
|   Deficiencies | Wernicke's encephalopathy |
| Infections | Systemic, CNS |
| Seizure | |
|   Postictal States | History of recent motor seizure |
|   Nonconvulsive status epilepticus | Seizure discharges on EEG |
| Stroke | |
|   Large hemisphere stroke | Associated focal findings |
|   Chronic subdural hematoma | Focal signs, elderly at highest risk, history of trauma |
| Post-anoxic encephalopathy | |
|   History of cardiac arrest | Myoclonus |
|   Ongoing hypoxia | Low oxygen saturation or $P_{O_2}$ |

## PAROXYSMAL EVENTS

| | |
|---|---|
| **Define paroxysmal symptoms.** | Symptoms that have a sudden onset and abrupt resolution |
| **What are four neurologic syndromes that cause paroxysmal manifestations?** | 1. Seizure<br>2. Migraine<br>3. Transient ischemic attack (TIA)<br>4. Syncope |
| **What clinical feature suggests a seizure?** | Abnormal, involuntary motor movements |
| **What two features suggest migraine?** | Headache<br>Scotomata |

| What two features suggest TIA? | Signs/symptoms in a vascular distribution<br>Suitable cardiogenic or vascular etiology |
|---|---|
| What clinical feature suggests vasomotor syncope (i.e., fainting)? | Autonomic manifestations, such as flushing, nausea, palpitations |
| Can syncope cause movements that look like convulsions? | Yes, but "convulsive syncope" is due to cerebral hypoperfusion and lacks the EEG changes of seizure. |

## PARKINSONISM AND PARKINSON'S DISEASE

| What is parkinsonism? | A set of signs and symptoms characterized by resting tremor, rigidity, and bradykinesia (slow movement), usually implying basal ganglia dysfunction |
|---|---|
| Distinguish Parkinson's disease from parkinsonism. | Parkinsonism is a set of signs and symptoms. Parkinson's disease is one of its causes and is histopathologically associated with Lewy body deposition. |
| Divide the clinical syndrome of parkinsonism into three etiologic groups. | 1. Idiopathic Parkinson's disease<br>2. Secondary parkinsonism (due to another identifiable cause)<br>3. Parkinson plus syndromes (associated with neurologic multisystem atrophies) |
| What two features distinguish secondary parkinsonism from idiopathic Parkinson's disease? | Those signs and symptoms associated with the various secondary causes and the identfication of a specific etiology |
| What is the most common cause of secondary parkinsonism? | Drugs, especially neuroleptic antipsychotics |
| What clinical features distinguish the Parkinson plus syndromes from idiopathic Parkinson's disease? | Signs of multisystem involvement of a Parkinson plus syndrome; these syndromes include progressive supranuclear palsy, Shy-Drager syndrome, and olivopontocerebellar degeneration |

| | |
|---|---|
| **What are some of these signs?** | Impairment of vertical downward gaze in progressive supranuclear palsy<br>Orthostatic hypotension and urinary incontinence in Shy-Drager syndrome<br>Cerebellar signs in olivopontocerebellar degeneration |
| **What is the difference in progression of symptoms between Parkinson plus syndromes and drug-induced parkinsonism?** | Symptoms in Parkinson plus syndromes progress gradually, whereas drug-induced parkinsonism is usually stable or monophasic. |
| **Which parkinsonian syndrome is most responsive to L-dopa?** | Idiopathic Parkinson's disease |

### Table 4–4.  Do-It-Yourself Differential Diagnosis of Parkinsonism

**Idiopathic**
  Parkinson's disease (Lewy bodies)

**Secondary Causes**
  Drugs (e.g., neuroleptics, including metoclopramide)
  Toxic (e.g., manganese, carbon monoxide, MPTP)
  Genetic (e.g., Wilson's disease, Hallervorden–Spatz disease, rigid Huntington's disease)
  Vascular (e.g., multi-infarct state)
  Neoplastic (e.g., frontal parasagittal tumors)

**Parkinson Plus Syndromes** (as part of a multisystem degenerative disorder)
  Progressive supranuclear palsy (Richardson–Steele–Olszewski syndrome)
  Progressive autonomic failure (Shy-Drager syndrome)
  Olivopontocerebellar degeneration

## TREMOR

| | |
|---|---|
| **What characteristic is most helpful in localizing the origin of tremor?** | The time at which the tremor occurs—whether the patient is at rest, making intentional movements, or maintaining posture |
| **What are two common causes of resting tremor?** | 1. Parkinson and related diseases (e.g., progressive supranuclear palsy, Shy-Drager syndrome)<br>2. Drugs that affect the basal ganglia (e.g., neuroleptic antipsychotics, neuroleptic antiemetics) |

| | |
|---|---|
| **What is the most common cause of intention tremor?** | Cerebellar disease |
| **What are two examples of "posture maintaining?"** | Holding the hands extended or holding the head erect |
| **What are four types of posture-maintaining tremor?** | Familial, adrenergic, physiologic, and essential |
| **What distinguishes familial tremor from the other types?** | Positive family history |
| **What causes adrenergic tremor?** | Adrenergic excess that may occur because of drugs (e.g., $\beta$-agonist bronchodilators) or metabolic abnormalities (e.g., hyperthyroidism) |
| **What is physiologic tremor?** | Posture-maintaining tremor associated with sustained muscle contraction or stress; it is normal |
| **What is essential tremor?** | It is the term used for posture-maintaining tremor when the tremor cannot be classified into the other categories. |
| **What is the name for essential tremor arising in the elderly?** | Senile tremor |

**Table 4–5.   Do-It-Yourself Differential Diagnosis of Tremor**

| When It Occurs | Etiology |
|---|---|
| Rest | Parkinson's and related diseases of basal ganglia |
| Intentional movement | Cerebellar disease |
| Posture maintenance | Familial or Essential<br>Adrenergic<br>Physiologic |

## DIZZINESS

| | |
|---|---|
| **What is dizziness?** | A general term that describes a variety of feelings, including vertigo, disequilibrium, and light-headedness or sensations that the patient interprets as abnormal. It has no specific pathophysiologic or localizing value. |
| **What is vertigo?** | A sense of rotational motion, indicating dysfunction of the vestibular pathways |
| **What is disequilibrium?** | A relatively specific term describing feeling "unsteady" or as though one is "about to fall," usually (but not exclusively) indicating an abnormal gait |
| **What is light-headedness?** | The sensation that one is about to faint |
| **What is a common cause of light-headedness?** | Presyncope |
| **What is presyncope?** | Transient cerebral hypoperfusion (as in orthostatic hypotension) |
| **What is syncope?** | Transient loss of consciousness of cardiovascular etiology; it is synonymous with fainting |
| **What is the importance of distinguishing among dizziness, vertigo, light-headedness and disequilibrium?** | Each one describes a different sensation, has different localizing value, and has different pathophysiologic implications. |
| **Localize peripheral and central vertigo by anatomic site.** | Peripheral—vestibular apparatus and vestibular nerve<br>Central—vestibular nucleus and pathways in brain stem |
| **Which is more common?** | Peripheral vertigo |
| **What are the three most common causes of peripheral vertigo?** | Benign paroxysmal positional vertigo (BPPV), labyrinthitis (also called vestibular neuronitis), Ménière's disease |

| | |
|---|---|
| **What distinguishes BPPV from other causes of vertigo?** | Vertigo is precipitated by specific movements of the head (i.e., it's positional) |
| **What are the three classic symptoms of Ménière's disease?** | Unilateral tinnitus, unilateral deafness, and paroxysmal vertigo |
| **What are three important causes of central vertigo?** | Vertebrobasilar TIA or stroke, brain stem tumor, CN VIII tumor |
| **What clinical feature distinguishes central from peripheral vertigo?** | Central vertigo is usually accompanied by other brain stem dysfunction. |
| **What two features distinguish peripheral from central vertigo?** | Tinnitus or unilateral deafness often accompany peripheral vertigo. |
| **Name four CNS locations where dysfunction can cause disequilibrium?** | 1. Whole brain (secondary either to primary CNS disorder of systemic illness)—focal or generalized weakness<br>2. Cerebellum—incoordination<br>3. Basal ganglia—impaired postural reflexes<br>4. Sensory tracts or receptors—impaired proprioception |
| **What symptoms help distinguish light-headedness caused by presyncope from disequilibrium?** | Presyncope may have transient autonomic symptoms. |

**Table 4–6.    Do-It-Yourself Differential Diagnosis of Dizziness**

| Symptom | Location | Clinical Significance |
|---|---|---|
| Disequilibrium | Basal ganglia | Impaired postural reflexes |
| | Cerebellum | Ataxia |
| | Sensory system | Loss of position sense (Proprioception) |
| | Diffuse CNS disease | Weakness, multifactorial |
| Vertigo | Peripheral | BPPV, labyrinthitis, Ménière's disease |
| | Central | Stroke, brain stem or CNS tumor |
| Light-headedness | Whole brain | Presyncope |

## ACUTE AND CHRONIC BACK PAIN (See also Chapter 12, Spine and Spinal Cord Disorders)

| | |
|---|---|
| Is most chronic back pain of neurologic or musculoskeletal origin? | Musculoskeletal |
| Cite the two most common locations of chronic back pain. | Upper (cervical) and lower (lumbosacral) back pain. |
| Name two pain-sensitive neurologic structures in the back. | Dura and posterior (sensory) nerve roots. |
| Name two common non-neurologic conditions causing chronic upper or lower back pain. | Para-vertebral muscle strain (myofascial pain) Degenerative (osteoarthritic) vertebral disease |
| How common is musculoskeletal low back pain? | It is the most common pain causing doctor visits. |
| What historical feature best distinguishes back pain of neurologic origin from musculoskeletal? | Lancinating pain in a dermatomal distribution |
| What physical examination finding best distinguishes back pain of neurologic origin from musculoskeletal? | An objective neurologic deficit on examination, such as an absent stretch reflex or weakness |
| State two events in the course of a patient with acute or chronic back pain that mandate an urgent search for structural spinal cord disease. | Onset of urinary incontinence or leg weakness |
| State two causes of intermittent leg claudication upon walking. | Peripheral vascular (arterial occlusive) disease to the legs Lumbosacral spinal canal stenosis with compression of the lower cord or roots |

**Define neuralgia.**

Paroxysmal pain radiating along one or more peripheral nerves

**State the most common cause of acute back pain with neuralgia.**

Herniated nucleus pulposus

## FOCAL WEAKNESS

**Localize the pathology that causes UMN signs.**

The motor system proximal to the anterior horn of the spinal cord (i.e., the corticospinal or corticobulbar tracts)

**Localize the pathology that causes LMN signs.**

The motor system at or distal to the anterior horn of the spinal cord (i.e., the motor nerve cell body and the peripheral nerves)

**What distribution of weakness distinguishes myopathic from neuropathic weakness?**

Myopathic weakness is usually proximal, whereas neuropathic weakness is usually distal either focal or generalized.

**What neurologic findings distinguish weakness caused by UMN lesions from LMN lesions?**

UMN: spasticity, hyperreflexia, Babinski's sign, clonus
LMN: hypotonia, hyporeflexia, muscle atrophy, fasciculations

**What is the distribution of weakness caused by lesions of motor cortex?**

Lateral motor cortex: contralateral hemiparesis; arm and face weaker than leg
Mesial motor cortex: contralateral hemiparesis; leg weaker than arm and face

**Of the internal capsule?**

Contralateral hemiparesis affecting the face, arm, and leg equally

**Of the spinal cord?**

Bilateral or unilateral weakness below level of lesion, sparing the face

**Of nerve root?**

Specific peripheral *and* paraspinal muscles supplied by the involved root

| | |
|---|---|
| **Of peripheral nerve?** | Specific peripheral muscles supplied by the involved nerve |
| **Of muscle?** | Diffuse weakness, usually proximal > distal |
| **What is the most proximal level of the neuraxis at which a lesion will cause LMN signs?** | LMN cell bodies in the brain stem or the anterior horn of the spinal cord |
| **What progressive disorder has both UMN and LMN signs?** | Amyotrophic lateral sclerosis (ALS), or Lou Gehrig's disease |
| **What are sensory findings in ALS?** | Normal—it only affects motor neurons |

## DIFFUSE WEAKNESS

| | |
|---|---|
| **What are the four levels of the peripheral motor system that, if affected, may cause weakness?** | 1. Anterior horn cell<br>2. Peripheral nerve<br>3. Neuromuscular junction<br>4. Muscle |
| **Name two levels where disease causes "neurogenic" weakness.** | Anterior horn cell or peripheral motor nerve |
| **What is the difference in distribution of neurogenic and myopathic weakness?** | Neurogenic: distal distribution<br>Myopathic: proximal distribution |
| **What are four causes of inflammatory myopathy?** | Polymyositis, dermatomyositis, inclusion body myositis, and infectious myositis (e.g., trichinosis) |
| **What are three causes of noninflammatory myopathy?** | Metabolic myopathies, congenital myopathies, and myoglobinuric myopathies |
| **What clinical characteristic distinguishes myoglobinuric from other myopathies?** | Symptoms are episodic and painful and are usually precipitated by exertion. |

| | |
|---|---|
| **Why are symptoms exertional?** | People with these diseases have defective muscle enzyme systems that fail when the muscles are used. |
| **What clinical characteristic distinguishes congenital from other myopathies?** | Congenital myopathies usually present at birth or in early childhood, although some present in adulthood. |
| **What is the difference between myopathy and muscular dystrophy (MD)?** | Myopathy is any disease affecting muscle. Dystrophy refers specifically to muscle diseases that cause loss of muscle cells, which are replaced by connective tissue and muscle atrophy. |
| **What are the two most common muscular dystrophies?** | Duchenne's and myotonic MD |
| **What are three other important muscular dystrophies?** | 1. Emery-Dreifuss MD<br>2. Facioscapulohumeral MD<br>3. Limb-girdle MD |
| **Which dystrophy is most likely to mimic motor neuron disease of childhood?** | Limb-girdle MD |
| **How is weakness distinguished from fatigue?** | Weakness is decreased muscle strength; fatigue is less precise and may describe lack of ability to sustain effort, subjective weariness, or sleepiness. |
| **What neuromuscular disorder characteristically has fatigable weakness?** | Myasthenia gravis |
| **What is fatigable weakness?** | Decreasing strength with persisting muscle contraction |
| **What distribution of myasthenic weakness distinguishes it from neurogenic and myopathic weakness?** | Early bulbar muscle weakness |

**Localize the muscle groups most severely affected in each of the following:**

| | |
|---|---|
| **Anterior horn cell disease?** | Distal muscle groups |
| **Peripheral neuropathy?** | Distal muscle groups |
| **Myasthenia gravis?** | Bulbar (cranial nerve) muscle groups |
| **Myopathy?** | Proximal muscle groups |

**Table 4–7.  Do-It-Yourself Differential Diagnosis of Myopathies**

| Type | Cause |
|---|---|
| Inflammatory | |
| Noninfectious | Polymyositis, dermatomyositis, inclusion body myopathy (IBM) |
| Infectious | Trichinosis |
| Noninflammatory | |
| Metabolic | Endocrine disorder (e.g., hypothyroidism) |
| | Enzyme defect (e.g., acid maltase deficiency) |
| | Mitochondrial disease (e.g., Kearns-Sayre; MERRF) |
| Congenital | Nemaline rod |
| | Central core |
| | Fiber-type disproportion |
| | Centronuclear (myotubular) |
| Myoglobinuric | Glycogen enzyme deficiency (e.g., McArdle's myophosphorylase) |
| | Glucose enzyme deficiency (e.g., phosphofructokinase) |
| | Lipid enzyme deficiency (e.g., carnitine palmityl transferase) |

**Table 4–8.**
**Do-It-Yourself Differential Diagnosis of Muscular Dystrophy**

| Onset of Weakness | Type |
|---|---|
| Childhood | Duchenne's, Emery-Dreifuss, Becker's, Congenital, limb-girdle, facioscapulohumeral |
| Adolescence | Myotonic, oculopharyngeal |

## PERIPHERAL NEUROPATHY (See also Chapter 13, Peripheral Nerve Disorders)

| | |
|---|---|
| **What is the most useful clinical characteristic for dividing peripheral neuropathies into groups?** | Progression of symptoms |

| | |
|---|---|
| **What are the three classes of peripheral neuropathies?** | Acute, subacute, and chronic |
| **Name three functional types of peripheral nerve fibers.** | Somatic motor, autonomic motor, and sensory |

## ACUTE NEUROPATHIES

| | |
|---|---|
| **Name an acute, exclusively sensory peripheral neuropathy?** | There are none |
| **What is the most significant and common type of acute motor peripheral neuropathy?** | Guillain-Barré syndrome |
| **What are two acute motor peripheral neuropathies that cause ascending weakness (i.e., those beginning in the distal extremities and progressing to muscles innervated by cranial nerves)?** | Guillain-Barré syndrome, porphyria |
|     **Two that cause descending weakness (i.e., those beginning in the cranial nerve–innervated muscles)?** | Miller-Fisher variant of Guillain-Barré syndrome, diphtheria |
| **What are two other neuromuscular disorders that usually begin with acute weakness of bulbar muscles (i.e., those innervated by cranial nerves)?** | Myasthenia gravis, botulism |

## SUBACUTE NEUROPATHIES

| | |
|---|---|
| **What is a sensorimotor peripheral neuropathy?** | A peripheral neuropathy involving both sensory and motor fibers |

| | |
|---|---|
| **What are the two most common causes of subacute sensorimotor peripheral neuropathy?** | Diabetes mellitus, alcohol |
| **What is the most common vitamin deficiency causing peripheral neuropathy?** | Vitamin $B_{12}$ deficiency |
| **What is an infectious cause of peripheral neuropathy, especially in tropical underdeveloped countries?** | Leprosy |
| **What type of cancer causes peripheral neuropathy by direct infiltration of nerves?** | Lymphoma |
| **What is the term for syndromes caused by the indirect effects, rather than direct invasion, of cancer?** | Paraneoplastic syndromes |
| **Can paraneoplastic syndromes cause peripheral neuropathy?** | Yes. They are especially associated with lung and visceral cancers. |

## CHRONIC NEUROPATHIES

| | |
|---|---|
| **Are most chronic peripheral neuropathies acquired or inherited?** | Inherited; they begin early in life |
| **What is the most common inherited peripheral neuropathy?** | Charcot-Marie-Tooth disease |
| **What are two other names for it?** | Hereditary motor-sensory neuropathy (HMSN) type 1<br>Peroneal muscular atrophy |
| **Is it the result of a systemic metabolic defect?** | No |

| | |
|---|---|
| **What is an inherited leukodystrophy that is caused by a systemic metabolic defect and accompanied by a peripheral neuropathy?** | Metachromatic leukodystrophy |
| **What clinical feature do all inherited peripheral neuropathies caused by a systemic metabolic defect have in common?** | All have other neurologic (and systemic) manifestations in addition to peripheral neuropathy, such as mental retardation in metachromatic leukodystrophy and Krabbe's disease |

### Table 4–9.
### Do-It-Yourself Differential Diagnosis of Peripheral Neuropathy

| Clinical Course | Comments |
|---|---|
| Acute motor peripheral neuropathy<br>    Guillain-Barré syndrome (GBS)<br>    Porphyria<br>    Diphtheria<br>    Miller-Fisher variant of GBS | |
| Subacute sensorimotor peripheral neuropathy (Acquired) | |
|     Toxic | Drugs (INH, nitrofurantoin, phenytoin, vinicristine) |
| | Toxins (alcohol, heavy metals, organophosphates, uremia) |
|     Metabolic | Endocrine disorder (diabetes, hypothyroidism) |
| | Deficiency [vitamin $B_{12}$ (pernicious anemia), thiamine (beriberi), niacin (pellagra)] |
|     Inflammatory | Infectious disease (leprosy) |
| | Autoimmune disorder (vasculitis, sarcoid) |
|     Neoplastic | Direct (lymphoma, amyloid, paraproteinemias) |
| | Paraneoplastic syndrome (antineuronal antibody associated) |
| Chronic sensorimotor peripheral neuropathy (Inherited) | |
|     Isolated peripheral neuropathy | Charcot-Marie-Tooth disease |
| | Dejerine-Sottas hypertrophic neuropathy |
| | Tomaculous peripheral neuropathy |
|     Peripheral neuropathy with other manifestations | Metachromatic leukodystrophy |
| | Refsum's disease (systemic metabolic defect) |
| | Abetalipoproteinemia, Tangier's disease |

| | |
|---|---|
| **What is C.I.D.P.?** | Chronic inflammatory demyelinating peripheral neuropathy |
| **What is its time course?** | Polyphasic; most other chronic neuropathies are continuous |

## NUMBNESS AND TINGLING

| | |
|---|---|
| **How do you distinguish if numbness and tingling originate from the brain, spinal cord, nerve root, or peripheral nerve?** | By the part of the body involved |
| **What distribution of symptoms suggests dysfunction in the brain?** | Hemisensory loss (arm and face or one half of body) |
| **In the spinal cord?** | A "sensory level" that coincides with a dermatomal level; below it sensation is impaired |
| **In the nerve root?** | Distribution of a single dermatome |
| **In a single peripheral nerve?** | Distribution of a single peripheral nerve (mononeuropathy) |
| **In diffuse peripheral nerves?** | "Stocking and glove" sensory loss (polyneuropathy) |
| **What is the term for pain of neural, especially peripheral nerve, origin?** | Neuralgia |
| **What is a common location for paresthesias associated with hyperventilation or anxiety?** | Perioral and bilateral fingers |
| **What is Lhermitte's sign?** | Electric-like sensation down the spine to the extremities when patient flexes head forward |
| **What is its basis?** | Stretching of posterior columns of the spinal cord or posterior nerve roots in patient with posterior spinal cord lesion |

**What is hypalgesia?**          The inability to feel painful sensation

**What is anesthesia?**          The inability to feel any sensation

**What is paresthesia?**         A "pins and needles" sensation

**What is hyperesthesia?**       Sensation that seems to be heightened

# 5

## Ethical and Legal Issues in Neurology (See also Chapter 21)

**State six ethical issues frequently encountered in neurologic practice.**

1. Determination of competence
2. Determination of capacity
3. Identification of surrogate
4. Informed consent
5. Termination of treatment
6. Certification of brain death

**What is competence?**

A legal judgment that may limit a person's rights

**What is capacity?**

Ability to make decisions

**How is capacity in medicine determined?**

Ask the patient to explain medical situation and choices.

**What are Advance Directives?**

Statements of treatment preferences made prior to incapacitation

**Name two common advance directives.**

Living Will and Durable Medical Power of Attorney

**What is a Living Will?**

Statement of interventions desired or rejected, usually at the end of life

**What is a Durable Medical Power of Attorney?**

Designation of a person to make health care decisions

**State two large groups of neurologic patients who merit advice on advance directives.**

Patients with progressing dementias or with motor neuron diseases (ALS, etc.)

**Who can make decisions for a patient who lacks medical decision-making capacity?**

Absent an advance directive, state law determines hierarchy of surrogate decision-makers

# Section II

Common
Neurologic
Conditions

# 6

# Headache and Facial Pain

**How common is headache?** More than 90% of the United States population had a headache in the past year.

**What best distinguishes an organic from a functional headache?** The presence of abnormalities on physical examination or on laboratory or imaging studies

**Which type is most common?** Functional headaches

**What are the three classes of functional headaches?**
1. Migraine headache
2. Tension (muscle contraction) headache
3. Chronic daily headache

## MIGRAINE HEADACHE

**What are three features of a classic migraine?**
1. Visual phenomena, especially scintillating scotomas
2. Nausea and/or vomiting
3. Hemicranial headache

**What are two features of a common migraine?**
1. Absence of visual phenomena
2. Bilateral headache, which is often periorbital or orbital

**What is the usual age of onset of migraines?** School-age or teenage

**What are five common migraine precipitants?** Alcohol, soft cheeses, bright lights or glare, chocolate, and sleep irregularity

**Anatomically localize the scintillating scotomata of migraine.** Occipital lobe

| | |
|---|---|
| **What drugs abort the headache of a migraine attack?** | Triptans, ergotamine tartrate |
| **What three classes of drugs prevent and/or reduce frequency of migraines?** | $\beta$-Blockers (e.g., propranolol) antiepilepsy drugs (e.g., valproate), tricyclics (e.g., amitriptyline) |
| **What is a complicated migraine?** | Migraine accompanied by a transient neurologic deficit |
| **What is the best treatment of childhood migraine?** | A nap (i.e., sleep it off) |

## TENSION (MUSCLE CONTRACTION) HEADACHE

| | |
|---|---|
| **What are the usual locations of a tension headache?** | Bilateral occipital, nuchal, frontal, or encircling the head |
| **What is the presumed cause of pain?** | Sustained cranial muscle contraction |
| **Are visual phenomena common?** | No |
| **Is nausea common?** | No–it is infrequent |
| **What is the best treatment?** | Oral analgesics that contain caffeine |
| **Another approach for Rx failures?** | Behavioral medicine, including biofeedback |

## OTHER HEADACHES

| | |
|---|---|
| **Describe chronic daily headache.** | Head pain all day every day |
| **Are analgesics effective treatment?** | No. Typically nothing helps. |
| **What is the treatment of choice?** | Eliminate analgesics; initiate tricyclics, such as amitriptyline. |
| **What is chronic paroxysmal hemicrania?** | Many daily short attacks of unilateral headache that last only minutes |

| | |
|---|---|
| **What is an effective treatment?** | Indomethacin |
| **What is cluster headache?** | Clustered attacks of orbital headache with nasal congestion and lacrimation |
| **Which gender is most affected?** | Males |
| **Usual time of onset?** | During sleep |
| **Distinguish the behavior of a person with cluster headache versus a person with migraine.** | A cluster patient paces; a migraine patient seeks solitude. |
| **What is the most frequent sequel of closed head injury?** | Headache |
| **Characterize the post-lumbar puncture (LP) headache.** | It intensifies when patient is erect and disappears when patient is prone. |
| **State the relationship, if any, between post-LP headache and:** | See also Chapter 30 |
| **Duration of rest after LP?** | None |
| **State of patient's hydration?** | None |
| **Bore of LP needle?** | The larger the bore, the greater the risk for headache. |
| **Number of LP attempts?** | The more the attempts, the greater the risk for headache. |
| **Characterize the pain of temporal arteritis.** | Throbbing; maximal over pulse of tender temporal artery |
| **What is a common lab finding in temporal arteritis?** | Elevated ESR |

| | |
|---|---|
| **What is a frequent associated systemic disorder?** | Polymyalgia rheumatica |
| **What is the treatment of temporal arteritis?** | Corticosteroids |
| **Why is temporal arteritis a relative emergency?** | If untreated, it may cause blindness because of involvement of arteries supplying the eye. |

## PSEUDOTUMOR CEREBRI

| | |
|---|---|
| **What distinguishes headache caused by elevated intracranial pressure from other headaches?** | Presence of papilledema and other focal neurologic signs |
| **What is a likely cause of headache when papilledema is present without a mass lesion?** | Pseudotumor cerebri (benign intracranial hypertension) |
| **Who gets it?** | Primarily young obese women |
| **How is it diagnosed?** | Elevated opening CSF pressure, but no mass lesion on imaging studies |
| **What additional symptom is important to detect?** | Deteriorating vision |
| **Why?** | Increased CSF pressure on the optic nerve may cause blindness. |
| **How should patients be followed?** | Regular examination of visual fields and acuity to detect deterioration |
| **How is it treated?** | Acetazolamide or surgical fenestration of the optic nerve sheath to release CSF |

## FACIAL PAIN

| | |
|---|---|
| **Describe trigeminal neuralgia.** | Paroxysmal, brief pain in the second and third divisions of the trigeminal cranial nerve (CN V) |

**What is another name for it?**

Tic douloureux

**Why is this a tic?**

The patient often winces from pain.

**What is its course?**

Usually recurrent for weeks

**What initiates a paroxysm?**

Sensory stimulus, such as touching the lip, smiling, chewing, shaving, etc.

**What class of drugs is used to treat it?**

Anticonvulsants (e.g., carbamazepine or phenytoin)

**What is the risk of using carbamazepine in elderly patients?**

Leukopenia

**What surgical procedure is used when medical management fails?**

Chemical ablation of the trigeminal sensory ganglion

**Localize temporomandibular joint (TMJ) pain.**

In front of the ear

**What are the typical causes?**

Trauma or arthritis of TMJ; malocclusion

**Therapy?**

Dental, surgical, or treat arthritis

**History question to ask patient's partner?**

Does the patient grind his/her teeth during sleep?

# 7        Stroke

## ISCHEMIC INFARCTION

**Define stroke.**

Death or damage of CNS tissue that has a vascular etiology

**What are the two major types of stroke?**

Ischemic and hemorrhagic stroke

**What are six treatable risk factors for stroke?**

Hypertension (HTN), heart disease, diabetes mellitus, cigarette smoking, alcohol abuse, and hyperlipidemia

**Is stroke more common in the brain or spinal cord?**

Brain

**Are most strokes of arterial or venous etiology?**

Arterial

**What is the clinical correlation between stroke manifestations and vascular anatomy?**

Stroke signs and symptoms point to a lesion of tissue nourished by a specific vascular system.

## VASCULAR ANATOMY

**What is the usual sequence of arteries in the left anterior circulation to the brain?**

Aorta, left common carotid, left internal carotid, left middle cerebral and left anterior cerebral arteries

**What is the usual sequence of arteries in the right anterior circulation to the brain?**

Aorta, innominate, right common carotid, right internal carotid, right middle cerebral and right anterior cerebral arteries

**Name three arteries that bring blood to the circle of Willis.**

1. Right internal carotid artery
2. Left internal carotid artery
3. Basilar artery

**Name the arteries of the circle of Willis.**

Right and left internal carotid arteries
Right and left middle cerebral arteries
Right and left anterior cerebral arteries
Anterior communicating artery
Right and left posterior communicating
    arteries
Right and left posterior cerebral
    arteries

**In the following figure, name each artery identified by letters *a* through *k*.**

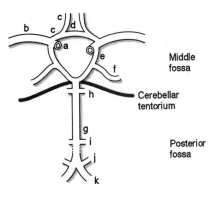

*a* = Internal carotid artery
*b* = Middle cerebral artery
*c* = Anterior cerebral artery
*d* = Anterior communicating artery
*e* = Posterior communicating artery
*f* = Posterior cerebral artery
*g* = Basilar artery
*h* = Superior cerebellar artery
*i* = Anterior inferior cerebellar artery
*j* = Posterior inferior cerebellar artery
    (PICA)
*k* = Vertebral artery

**Which circle of Willis artery is most often vestigial?**

A posterior communicating artery

**Which is most often reduplicated?**

An anterior communicating artery

**Is the circle of Willis usually functionally complete or incomplete?**

Incomplete

**Where do aneurysms occur in the circle of Willis?**

Aneurysms usually occur at bifurcations.

**What are the three largest branches of the vertebrobasilar system?**

1. Posterior inferior cerebellar artery (PICA)
2. Anterior inferior cerebellar artery
3. Superior cerebellar artery

**What is the usual origin of the:**

    **Lenticulostriate arteries?**

Proximal middle cerebral artery

    **Anterior choroidal artery?**

Internal carotid artery opposite orifice of middle cerebral

    **PICA?**

Vertebral artery

    **Anterior spinal artery?**

Vertebral arteries

**Which of these arteries is Charcot's "artery of apoplexy?"**

Lenticulostriate artery

**Are there usually one or more than one lenticulostriate?**

Usually several in each hemisphere

**What systemic illness predisposes these arteries to rupture (apoplexy)?**

HTN

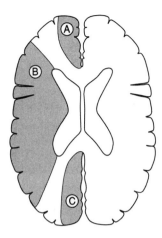

| What symptoms result from its occlusion on the right? | Left hemibody sensory loss, neglect, and hemiparesis |
| What symptoms result from its occlusion on the left? | Aphasia, right hemiparesis |
| What is the vascular territory of the anterior cerebral artery? | Anterior medial hemisphere |
| What is the vascular territory of the middle cerebral artery? | Most of the cerebral hemisphere, except small medial areas served by the anterior and posterior cerebral arteries |
| Which letter represents this in the diagram? | B |

| | |
|---|---|
| **Which letter represents this in the diagram?** | A |
| **What symptoms result from its occlusion?** | Contralateral leg weakness |
| **What is the vascular territory of the posterior cerebral artery?** | Posterior medial hemisphere |
| **Which letter represents this in the diagram?** | C |
| **What symptoms result from its occlusion?** | Contralateral hemianopia without paralysis |
| **Why is the edge of each vascular territory spared from infarction?** | A "watershed" area receives overlap in arterial supply |
| **What causes watershed infarction?** | Hypotension, which does not provide enough cerebral perfusion pressure for blood to reach end arterioles |
| **What is the vascular territory of the vertebrobasilar arteries?** | Brain stem (i.e., medulla, pons, midbrain) and cerebellum |
| **What is lateral medullary infarction or Wallenberg Syndrome?** | A very complex stroke syndrome, it consists of brain stem and cerebellar manifestations, without arm or leg paralysis or altered consciousness. |
| **Where is it located?** | It is located in the lower brain stem (medulla). |
| **How is it caused?** | It is due to ischemia of the lateral medulla, which is nourished by the posterior inferior cerebellar artery, which originates from the vertebral. |

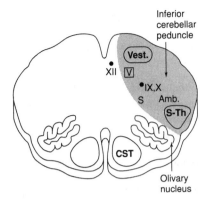

*CST*: corticospinal tract in pyramid; *Amb*: nucleus ambiguus (IX and X); S: descending sympathetic pathway from hypothalamus to T-1; *vest*: vestibular nucleus; V: descending (spinal) nucleus C.N.V.; *S-Th*: ascending lateral spinothalamic tract.

**The figure shows a cross-section of the medulla. What artery supplies the shaded area in the diagram?**

PICA (posterior inferior cerebellar artery) originating from the ipsilateral vertebral artery

**What other brain region does it supply?**

Medial cerebellar hemisphere

**List the findings of a lateral medullary infarction (Wallenberg's syndrome):**
  **Autonomic?**

Ipsilateral Horner's syndrome from involvement of descending autonomic fibers (s)

  **Motor?**

None. The corticospinal tracts are spared because they are in the *medial* medulla (CST).

  **Cranial nerve?**

Dysarthria, dysphagia, vertigo, and nystagmus (IX, X, vestibular)

  **Sensory?**

Diminished pain and temperature of the *ipsilateral* face (trigeminal nucleus) and *contralateral* body (crossed spinothalamic tracts) (V and S-Th)

| | |
|---|---|
| **Coordination?** | Ipsilateral cerebellar incoordination |
| **Occlusion of which artery causes coma?** | Basilar |
| **Which vessels are usually responsible for the locked-in syndrome of vascular etiology?** | Basilar artery branches to the base of the pons |
| **What pupillary abnormality often accompanies dissection of the extracranial internal carotid artery?** | Miosis (Horner's syndrome) secondary to injury to the sympathetic nerve in the carotid sheath |

## CLASSIFICATION OF STROKES BY VESSEL SIZE

| | |
|---|---|
| **Why should strokes be distinguished as large or small vessel strokes?** | Because they differ in pathophysiology of stenosis, clinical presentation, risk factors, and therapy |
| **What six arteries are affected in large vessel strokes?** | The five vessels of the circle of Willis (ICA, MCA, ACA, PCA, basilar) as well as the vertebral arteries |
| **What arteries are affected in small vessel strokes?** | Small unnamed arteries that arise from all of the large branches of the circle of Willis |
| **What is the typical pathology of large and small vessel occlusion?** | **Large vessel**—atheromatous embolic disease<br>**Small vessel**—lipohyalinosis |
| **How are large and small vessel strokes distinguished clinically?** | Large vessel strokes affect large areas of brain, often whole lobes, whereas small vessel strokes affect small areas |

## LARGE VESSEL ISCHEMIC STROKE

| | |
|---|---|
| **What are the three most frequent causes?** | 1. Cardiogenic embolization<br>2. Arteriogenic embolization<br>3. In situ arterial thrombosis |
| **What are four conditions that predispose a person to cardiogenic embolization?** | 1. Atrial fibrillation<br>2. Dilated cardiomyopathy<br>3. Valvular disease<br>4. Endocardial damage caused by myocardial infarction |

**Identify the most common condition predisposing to arteriogenic cerebral embolization and its location.**

Atheromatous deposition in the carotid sinus area, just above carotid artery bifurcation

**Do carotid artery stenosis and endothelial ulceration often coexist?**

Yes

**What is the classic physical sign of carotid artery stenosis/ulceration?**

Carotid bruit

**Describe a carotid bruit.**

A murmur that is loudest over the artery not transmitted up from the heart

**What is another name for a carotid Doppler directional blood flow study?**

A noninvasive carotid evaluation, or **NICE** study

**What three studies best evaluate the carotid artery as a cause of ischemic stroke?**

NICE study, carotid angiography, magnetic resonance angiography (MRA)

**What is the treatment of moderate-to-severe (65%–99%) carotid stenosis in a symptomatic patient?**

Carotid endarterectomy

**What procedure best evaluates the heart as a source of cerebral embolization?**

Transthoracic or transesophageal echocardiography

**What is the best treatment in an asymptomatic carotid stenosis?**

Uncertain. Probably nothing or taking one aspirin daily. Some recent studies support carotid endarterectomy for severe stenosis. Outcome from surgical intervention depends on the surgeon's experience and track record.

**Define the following varieties of ischemic stroke:**
    **Transient ischemic attack (TIA)?**

Deficits reverse in less than 24 hours

**Stroke in progress (evolving stroke)?**

Deficits evolve while the patient is under observation

**Reversible ischemic neurologic deficit (RIND)?**

Deficits reverse or essentially reverse in more than 24 hours

**Completed stroke?**

Deficits remain

**Describe the typical course of an ischemic stroke.**

Abrupt onset of deficits, followed by plateau, followed by improvement to or toward normal

**Why may manifestations of a massive ischemic stroke continue to worsen for 24–36 hours after onset?**

Because of local edema secondary to damage to CNS cells

**What is the role of anticoagulation in ischemic stroke?**

It is *indicated* for patients with a known thromboembolic source in the heart. It is *usually indicated* in patients at risk for cardiogenic embolization, such as those with atrial fibrillation or dilated cardiomyopathy. It *may be useful* for patients who continue to have TIAs despite antiplatelet agents or who are having a stroke in progress.

**What is a contraindication to anticoagulation?**

Large hemispheric stroke that is more liable to bleed

**What is the role of antiplatelet agents in ischemic stroke?**

Secondary prevention of stroke

**Name three antiplatelet agents useful for secondary prevention of stroke.**

Aspirin, clopidogrel (Plavix), ticlopidine (Ticlid), aspirin-dipyridamole combination (Aggrenox)

**What potential side effect is shared by all?**

Bleeding risks

**What are important potential side effects of ticlopidine?**

Hematologic: neutropenia/agranulocytosis (1–2%), aplastic anemia (1:4,000), thrombotic thrombocytopenic purpura, TTP (1:2,000), which prevent its use except when benefit outweighs the risk.

| | |
|---|---|
| **What rare important side effect of clopidogrel necessitates monitoring?** | TTP (8 per million) |
| **What are the first emergency department steps after an acute stroke?** | **ABC**—airway, breathing, circulation |
| **What is the second emergency department step?** | Head CT scan to rule out intracranial hemorrhage |
| **How is blood pressure managed?** | Avoid excessive reduction; tolerate mild hypertension |

## SMALL VESSEL ISCHEMIC STROKE

| | |
|---|---|
| **What term identifies a small infarct after occlusion of a small artery?** | A lacune, or small vessel stroke |
| **What are two risk factors for lacunar infarcts?** | HTN, diabetes mellitus |
| **What are four common sites for lacunar infarcts?** | 1. Internal capsule<br>2. Thalamus<br>3. Basal ganglia<br>4. Pons |
| **Can lacunar infarcts be clinically silent?** | Yes |
| **Can lacunar infarcts cause localized and limited signs and symptoms?** | Yes |
| **Can an accumulation of lacunar infarcts gradually produce signs and symptoms?** | Yes |
| **What may distinguish hemiparesis caused by a small vessel stroke from that caused by a large vessel stroke?** | Small vessel stroke: no sensory loss; equal weakness in face, arm, and leg<br>Large vessel stroke: sensory deficit; face and arm affected more than leg |

**Why?**

The small vessel stroke, or lacune, damages a small area, usually in the motor pathway of internal capsule or pons and misses sensory paths; whereas a large vessel stroke (e.g., an MCA) damages the frontal motor cortex serving the face and arm plus the parietal sensory cortex. The leg area of cortex is spared because it is in ACA territory.

**What distinguishes sensory loss caused by a small vessel stroke from that caused by a large vessel stroke?**

Small vessel stroke in thalamus is not associated with motor deficits, whereas large vessel stroke of MCA causes both motor and sensory losses.

**Why?**

Small vessel stroke in thalamus misses motor pathways (corticospinal tracts). Large vessel stroke includes the motor pathways.

**What term describes the motor effects of multiple lacunar infarcts scattered through the brain and brain stem?**

Pseudobulbar palsy

**What are the two most prominent features of pseudobulbar palsy?**

Spastic speech and swallowing; emotional incontinence (pathologic emotionality)

**What is pseudobulbar emotionality?**

Crying or laughing that is not proportional to the emotional content of the stimulus

**What is the pathophysiologic basis of pseudobulbar emotionality?**

Disruption of corticobulbar UMNs to brain stem nuclei

**Name two motor accompaniments.**

Hyperactive jaw jerk; slowed spastic tongue movements (Often: grasp, snout, or glabellar reflexes also)

**What is the MRI picture?**

Multifocal areas of increased T2 signal intensity

**With what disease is this most easily confused?**

MS

| | |
|---|---|
| **What term describes the cognitive effects of multiple lacunar infarcts scattered through the brain?** | Multi-infarct dementia |

## INTRACEREBRAL HEMORRHAGE (ICH)

| | |
|---|---|
| **Which stroke is more common, a subarachnoid hemorrhage or ICH?** | ICH |
| **What two racial groups have a high rate of hypertensive ICH?** | Asians and African Americans |
| **Name four major risk factors for ICH.** | 1. HTN<br>2. Low serum cholesterol<br>3. Aspirin therapy<br>4. Anticoagulation therapy |
| **Name five important causes.** | 1. HTN<br>2. Amyloid angiopathy<br>3. Metastatic tumors<br>4. Vasculitis<br>5. Illicit drugs |
| **Name three major cerebral complications of ICH.** | Edema, herniation, and rebleeding |
| **Where are the four most common sites in the brain for hypertensive ICH?** | Putamen, thalamus, cerebellum, and pons |
| **What is the classic location of ICH associated with HTN?** | Basal ganglia (rather than the cortex) |
| **What is the most common cause of ICH involving an entire brain lobe in the elderly?** | Cerebral amyloid angiopathy |
| **Cerebral amyloid angiopathy is confirmed by histopathologic evaluation and positive staining with which dye?** | Congo red dye causes birefringence when viewed under polarized light. |

**Is cerebral amyloid angiopathy associated with systemic vascular amyloidosis?**

No

**Is ICH due to cerebral amyloid angiopathy associated with HTN?**

No

**What histopathologic changes are in the microvasculature of individuals who suffer a hypertensive ICH?**

Lipohyalinosis; segmental fibrinoid degeneration; microaneurysm (saccular or fusiform)

**Name the four metastatic tumors to the brain that are most frequently associated with ICH.**

**M**elanoma
**C**horiocarcinoma
**R**enal cell carcinoma
**B**ronchogenic carcinoma
(Mnemonic: **My Cat Really Bleeds**)

**What is the primary brain neoplasm most commonly associated with ICH?**

Glioblastoma multiforme

**What three brain CT findings characterize ICH due to metastatic neoplasms?**

Multiple lesions; large amount of edema; ring enhancement with contrast

**Does oral anticoagulation increase risk of ICH?**

Yes, by about 10-fold

**Is primary CNS vasculitis commonly associated with systemic symptoms?**

No

**What is the appearance of CNS vasculitis on angiography?**

'String of beads" appearance from multiple dilatations and constrictions

**Does vasculitis of cerebral arteries usually cause ICH or ischemic cerebral infarction?**

Ischemic cerebral infarction

| | |
|---|---|
| **What illicit drug is most commonly associated with ICH?** | Cocaine |
| **ICH is the presenting feature in what percent of patients with vascular malformations?** | 50% |
| **What is the brain CT image of an acute ICH?** | A bright circular object within the brain parenchyma |
| **What is the brain MRI image of an acute ICH?** | Normal or low signal on $T_1$<br>Low signal on $T_2$ surrounded by increased signal of edema |
| **What is believed to be the cause of decreased level of consciousness in most patients with ICH?** | Increased intracranial pressure |
| **Does the absence of headache and vomiting upon presentation with an acute focal neurologic deficit make ICH less likely?** | No |
| **What is the cause of ischemic infarcts that develop after an ICH?** | Local mass effect produced by the hematoma and edema |
| **In what brain location does an ICH cause recurrent seizures?** | Cortex |
| **Why is a cerebellar hemorrhage a surgical emergency?** | Early surgical resection prevents brain stem herniation and prognosis for recovery of cerebellar function is excellent, even with large resections. |
| **What is the major predictor of morbidity and mortality of hypertensive ICH?** | Size of the hematoma |
| **What is the overall mortality of hypertensive ICH?** | 40% |

## SUBARACHNOID HEMORRHAGE (SAH)

**What is the most frequent cause of SAH?**

Head trauma

**What is the name of nontraumatic subarachnoid bleeding?**

Primary SAH

**What is the most common etiology of primary SAH?**

Ruptured cerebral aneurysm

**What percent of patients die within 24 hours of onset of SAH?**

Approximately 25%, but prognosis depends on the grade (severity) of SAH at presentation

**The highest incidence of SAH occurs in which decades of life?**

Fourth, fifth, and sixth decades

**Name two morphologic types of cerebral aneurysms based on radiographic appearance.**

Saccular and fusiform

**Most aneurysms are of what type?**

Saccular

**What are two synonyms for *saccular* aneurysm?**

Berry, or congenital, aneurysm

**Are these aneurysms present at birth?**

No. A defect in the media of the arterial wall is present. The aneurysm develops later.

**The term *mycotic aneurysm* implies what type of etiology?**

Infectious—a true mycotic aneurysm implies a fungal etiology

**Do most cerebral aneurysms occur in the anterior or posterior circulation?**

Anterior circulation

**Where do most saccular aneurysms specifically occur within the cerebral vasculature?**

At the bifurcation of the large cerebral arteries at the base of the skull (circle of Willis) or first division of middle cerebral artery in Sylvian fissure

**Name the four hallmark symptoms of rupture.**

Headache, syncope, nausea, and vomiting

**What is the defining characteristic of the headache?**

Abrupt, severe headache; "the worst headache of my life"

**What are prodromal or warning symptoms before major aneurysmal rupture?**

Severe headache, especially focal pain behind the eyes (retroorbital pain) and/or a stiff neck from leakage of a small amount of blood ("sentinel hemorrhage")

**What cranial nerve abnormalities should raise the suspicion of an aneurysm of the posterior communicating artery?**

Third-nerve palsy with diminished light reflex and pupillary dilation

**What does initial emergency evaluation for suspected SAH include?**

Noncontrasted brain CT and, if SAH is noted, a cerebral angiogram

**If SAH is suspected and brain CT reveals no hemorrhage, what should be done?**

Lumbar puncture for CSF to examine for hemorrhage (increased RBC)

**List three features of the CSF that help distinguish SAH from a "traumatic tap."**

1. Equal RBC count in first and third tubes
2. Xanthochromic color after CSF centrifugation
3. Crenation of RBCs

**Why isn't MRI the diagnostic test of choice for acute SAH?**

Because acute SAH cannot always be distinguished from normal CSF on MRI

**What are the four initial laboratory tests for the evaluation of SAH?**

Electrolytes, CBC, ECG, and blood cultures

**Why is each test obtained?**

**Electrolytes**—to check the sodium level, which may be low because of SIADH

**CBC**—to check the hematocrit; if elevated, it may increase the risk of ischemia
**ECG**—may be transiently abnormal
**Blood cultures**—if a mycotic aneurysm is suspected

**What does acute management of SAH include?**

Bed rest, stool softeners, quiet environment, elevation of the head of the bed and control of HTN, all of which help reduce blood pressure in the aneurysm; calcium channel antagonists (e.g., nimodipine) reduce vasospasm

**What is the definitive treatment of SAH from ruptured aneurysm?**

Early surgical repair by clipping the aneurysm

**What are four complications of ruptured aneurysm that cause subsequent neurologic deficits?**

Cerebral ischemia from vasospasm; acute hydrocephalus from clot; bleeding from rerupture; increased risk of future development of normal pressure hydrocephalus

**What is the *major* cause of delayed morbidity and mortality?**

Cerebral ischemia due to vasospasm

**What are clinical symptoms of cerebral vasospasm?**

Decreased consciousness with or without focal signs (e.g., hemiparesis)

**How is cerebral vasospasm managed?**

Hypertensive hypervolemic therapy (HHT), cerebral artery angioplasty, vasodilators (e.g., papaverine)

**How many days post-SAH is cerebral vasospasm most likely to occur?**

3–10 days following the initial hemorrhage

# 8

# Seizures and Epilepsy

## DEFINITIONS

| | |
|---|---|
| **What is a seizure?** | Temporary alteration of brain function caused by paroxysmal, abnormal cerebral neuronal discharge |
| **What is an ictus?** | A seizure |
| **What is a convulsion?** | A seizure causing abnormal muscle contractions |
| **What is epilepsy?** | Continuing tendency to spontaneous recurrent seizures, resulting from a persistent pathologic process |
| **What is a seizure disorder?** | Synonymous with epilepsy |
| **What is a provoked seizure?** | A seizure occurring in an otherwise normal brain as a result of some transient alteration, such as changes in glucose or sodium or drug effects. |
| **What is status epilepticus?** | Continuing or recurring seizures without return of normal consciousness (see Chapter 17) |

## SEIZURE TYPES

| | |
|---|---|
| **What is the most common type of seizure?** | Complex partial seizures |
| **On what basis are seizures classified?** | They are classified according to observable clinical manifestations by the International League Against Epilepsy (ILAE). |
| **What are the two main categories of seizures?** | Generalized and partial (focal) seizures |

| | |
|---|---|
| **What is the defining clinical difference between generalized and partial seizures?** | Consciousness is lost in generalized seizures and preserved in partial seizures. |
| **What is the pathophysiologic significance of this?** | Preservation of consciousness implies seizures arise from an area of *localized* pathology. |
| **Name two categories of seizures that may make the patient unable to respond to questions.** | Generalized seizures and complex partial seizures |

## PARTIAL SEIZURES

| | |
|---|---|
| **What is another name for partial seizures?** | Focal seizures |
| **What are the subdivisions of partial seizures?** | Simple partial seizure and complex partial seizure |
| **What characteristic distinguishes simple partial from complex partial seizures?** | Consciousness is normal in simple partial seizures. In complex partial seizures, consciousness is impaired (i.e., patients are awake but not normally interactive with the environment). |

## SIMPLE PARTIAL SEIZURES

| | |
|---|---|
| **How are simple partial seizures further subdivided?** | Based on whether symptoms are primarily motor, sensory, autonomic, or psychic |
| **Describe the following types of simple partial seizures:** | |
| **Simple partial motor seizure** | Repetitive jerking of a body part (e.g., face, arm, or leg) |
| **Simple partial sensory seizure** | Tingling of a body region |
| **Autonomic partial seizure** | Abdominal or epigastric sensations, often poorly described as a "rising" sensation |

| | |
|---|---|
| **Psychic simple partial seizure** | Auditory, visual, gustatory, or olfactory illusions; déjà vu; jamais vu |
| **What is déjà vu?** | Feeling as though something has been seen or experienced before; literal French translation is "already seen" |
| **What is jamais vu?** | Feeling of unfamiliarity in a familiar situation; literal French translation is "never seen" |
| **What is an aura?** | A simple partial seizure occurring as the prelude to a more widespread seizure; the focal start of a seizure |
| **What is the significance of an aura?** | It occurs only in seizures with a focal onset and may help localize the site of seizure onset. |

## COMPLEX PARTIAL SEIZURES

| | |
|---|---|
| **Describe a typical complex partial seizure.** | Impaired alertness and responsiveness with amnesia for the events; sometimes preceded by an aura and followed by a postictal state |
| **What are possible objective accompaniments to a complex partial seizure?** | Confused purposeless behavior (automatisms), especially lip smacking, vocalizations, swallowing, and fumbling |
| **What is a postictal state?** | Temporary postseizure neurologic deficit (most commonly lethargy), possibly secondary to neuronal exhaustion |
| **What is Todd's paralysis?** | A postictal state consisting of transient hemiparesis, reflecting the location of the most involved area of the brain |
| **Name a seizure that originates in one brain area and subsequently spreads throughout the brain.** | Partial seizure with secondary generalization |

## GENERALIZED SEIZURES

**Name seven types of generalized seizure.**

1. Generalized tonic-clonic (GTC; formerly called grand mal) seizure
2. Absence seizure (formerly called petit mal)
3. Myoclonic seizure
4. Tonic seizure
5. Clonic seizure
6. Atonic seizure
7. Infantile spasm

**Describe the essential features of a GTC seizure.**

Sudden generalized stiffness that lasts a few seconds during the tonic phase, followed by rhythmic muscle contractions during the clonic phase, followed by postictal somnolence or confusion; it is truly a GTC seizure only when both tonic and clonic phases are present

**What are other common accompanying symptoms?**

Injury during falling, tongue biting, stertorous respirations, urinary incontinence, and drooling

**Describe the essential features of an absence seizure.**

Sudden staring unresponsiveness that lasts a few to several seconds and interrupts ongoing activities, with resumption of activity immediately on termination of the seizure.

**What are other common accompanying symptoms?**

If it is prolonged, it may be accompanied by automatisms, similar to a complex partial seizure.

**Describe a myoclonic seizure.**

A single, sudden, lightening-like jerk of the whole body or a group of muscles, which may cause the patient to drop or throw something held in the hand (e.g., a fork while eating)

**Name an epilepsy syndrome in which myoclonic seizures are common.**

Juvenile myoclonic epilepsy (JME)

**Describe a clonic seizure.**

Rhythmic muscle contractions, identical to the clonic phase of a GTC seizure

| | |
|---|---|
| **How does a clonic seizure differ from a myoclonic seizure?** | Clonic seizures are multiple rhythmic jerks, whereas myoclonic seizures are single jerks, although several may occur in sequence arrhythmically. |
| **Describe a tonic seizure.** | Sudden, sustained, whole body muscle contraction that lasts several seconds; typically the extremities, back, and neck are pulled into extension |
| **Describe an atonic seizure.** | Sudden loss of whole body muscle tone, associated with falling limp to the ground; consciousness usually returns quickly |
| **Name a childhood epilepsy syndrome in which atonic seizures are common.** | Lennox-Gastaut syndrome |
| **Describe an infantile spasm.** | Sudden contraction of the trunk and arms, flexing the trunk forward and pulling the arms into extension; also called a "salaam" attack |
| **Name a childhood epilepsy syndrome in which infantile spasms are common.** | West's syndrome |

**Outline an algorithm for classifying seizure types.**

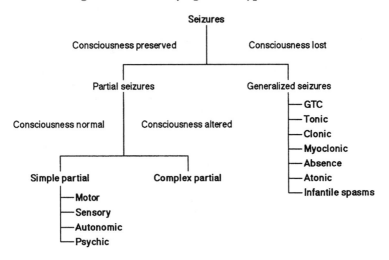

## EPILEPSY SYNDROMES

What is the difference between *seizures* and *epilepsy syndromes?*

Seizures are symptoms and signs. Epilepsy syndromes are diseases.

What is the advantage of using epilepsy syndromes, rather than only seizure type, to characterize patients?

It is more informative. Patients with a given epilepsy syndrome have a similar natural history, response to treatment, and presumably share the same pathophysiology.

What is the prevalence of epilepsy?

As much as 10% of the population experiences a seizure sometime in life, but only about 3–5% of the population has epilepsy.

| **How are epilepsy syndromes categorized into groups by the ILAE classification?** | They are fundamentally based on whether a focal (also called partial or localization-related) or a generalized pathologic process is present and also whether the process is idiopathic, symptomatic, or cryptogenic (Table 8-1). |

### Table 8–1.    Reference Table of ILAE Epilepsy Syndromes

| Category | Focal | Generalized |
|---|---|---|
| Idiopathic | BREC<br>Childhood epilepsy with occipital paroxysms | Benign neonatal convulsions<br>Benign myoclonic epilepsy in infancy<br>Childhood absence epilepsy<br>Juvenile absence epilepsy<br>JME<br>Epilepsy with GTCs on awakening<br>Reflex epilepsy (e.g., primary reading epilepsy) |
| Symptomatic | TLE, such as mesial (amygdalohippocampal) and lateral temporal (neocortical)<br>Frontal lobe<br>Parietal lobe<br>Occipital lobe<br>Rasmussen's encephalitis<br>Most reflex epilepsies | Early myoclonic encephalopathy<br>Early infantile epileptic encephalopathy with suppression-burst<br>Cortical abnormalities (e.g., malformations, dysplasias)<br>Metabolic abnormalities |
| Cryptogenic | Any occurrence of partial seizures with suspected histopathology | West's syndrome<br>Lennox-Gastaut syndrome<br>Epilepsy with myoclonic-astatic seizures<br>Epilepsy with myoclonic absences |

BREC, childhood absence epilepsy, JME, TLE, West's syndrome, and Lennox-Gastaut syndrome are discussed in Chapter 8.
BREC = benign rolandic epilepsy of childhood; GTC = general tonic–clonic; JME = juvenile myoclonic epilepsy; TLE = temporal lobe epilepsy.

| **Describe the general difference between symptomatic, cryptogenic, and idiopathic epilepsy syndromes.** | **Symptomatic epilepsies** result from a known histopathologic abnormality in the brain.<br>**Cryptogenic epilepsies** presumably have a structural basis because of their association with other neurologic symptoms, but that basis is not known. |

**Idiopathic epilepsies** usually are inherited and presumably are due to abnormalities of neurotransmission without associated structural abnormalities.

**On what five characteristics is an epilepsy syndrome based?**

1. Type of seizure
2. EEG
3. Age at onset
4. Interictal neurologic abnormalities
5. Natural history

**What is the most common epilepsy syndrome?**

Temporal lobe epilepsy (TLE)

## TLE

**Is TLE a partial or generalized epilepsy syndrome?**

Partial

**What is the main seizure type present in this syndrome?**

Complex partial seizures

**What is the most common interictal EEG finding?**

Spikes or sharp waves originating in the temporal region of the head

**What is the most common associated MRI abnormality?**

Atrophy and high T2 signal intensity of the hippocampus and other mesial temporal lobe structures; another term for this type of TLE is mesial temporal lobe epilepsy

**What is the most common histopathologic finding in the temporal lobe?**

Mesial temporal sclerosis, consisting of neuronal loss and gliosis in the hippocampus

## BENIGN ROLANDIC EPILEPSY OF CHILDHOOD (BREC)

**What type of epilepsy syndrome is BREC?**

Idiopathic focal epilepsy

**Who gets BREC?**

Children

**Why is it considered benign?**

Seizures almost universally abate in adolescence.

| | |
|---|---|
| **What is the classic EEG finding?** | Spikes in the centrotemporal region of the head, which is why the ILEA name is *benign childhood epilepsy with centrotemporal spikes*. The Rolandic area is around the central sulcus, which contains the primary motor cortex. |
| **Describe a typical seizure due to BREC.** | Simple motor seizure arising in the face region of the motor cortex, consisting of drooling, inability to speak, and clonic facial movements. It may secondarily generalize into a convulsion. |

## CHILDHOOD ABSENCE EPILEPSY

| | |
|---|---|
| **What type of epilepsy syndrome is childhood absence epilepsy?** | Idiopathic generalized epilepsy |
| **What is the classic EEG finding?** | Generalized 3-Hz spike and wave |
| **How long does childhood absence epilepsy persist?** | It usually abates in adolescence. |

## JME

| | |
|---|---|
| **What type of epilepsy syndrome is JME?** | Idiopathic generalized epilepsy |
| **What are the two main types of seizures accompanying JME?** | Myoclonic jerks and generalized clonic seizures |
| **What is the classic EEG finding?** | Generalized multiple-spike and wave |

## LENNOX-GASTAUT SYNDROME

| | |
|---|---|
| **What type of epilepsy syndrome is Lennox-Gastaut syndrome?** | Cryptogenic generalized epilepsy, because it is associated with static encephalopathy but the offending histopathology is not identifiable. |

| | |
|---|---|
| **What are its two main clinical characteristics?** | Static encephalopathy (mental retardation) and seizures beginning in childhood |
| **How long does Lennox-Gastaut syndrome persist?** | Throughout life |
| **What is the classic EEG finding?** | Slow spike and wave; it is slow because it is less than 3 Hz |

## WEST'S SYNDROME

| | |
|---|---|
| **What type of epilepsy syndrome is West's syndrome?** | Cryptogenic generalized epilepsy |
| **What is West's syndrome?** | Infantile spasms occurring with developmental delay and a hypsarrhythmia EEG pattern |
| **What is the difference between infantile spasms and West's syndrome?** | Infantile spasms refer only to a type of seizure that may occur in different epilepsy syndromes. West's syndrome refers specifically to infantile spasms occurring with developmental delay. |
| **How long does West's syndrome persist?** | Infantile spasms abate in early childhood, but static encephalopathy and other seizure types persist throughout life. |

## CHILDHOOD FEBRILE SEIZURES

| | |
|---|---|
| **Who gets them?** | Otherwise normal children "between the 6's" (6 months to 6 years) |
| **Characterize a simple febrile seizure.** | Single, short generalized tonic-clonic convulsion during a fever |
| **Should they receive A.E.D's?** | Only if it is a complex febrile seizure |
| **Define complex febrile seizure.** | Longer than 30 minutes or any focal features |

## PSEUDOSEIZURE

**What is a pseudoseizure?**

A nonepileptic event mimicking an electroconvulsive seizure

**Name some events that could be considered a pseudoseizure.**

Hysterical behavior, conversion reaction, malingering, learned behavior

## DIAGNOSTIC TESTS

**Is EEG indicated in the evaluation of seizures?**

Yes, for almost all patients

**Why?**

To distinguish partial from generalized seizure disorders

To localize site of seizure onset in partial seizures

To characterize the epilepsy syndrome (see Chapter 46)

**What is the characteristic EEG abnormality in seizure disorders?**

Spikes and sharp waves

**What is the difference between a spike and a sharp wave?**

A spike is more pointed, because it is shorter in duration.

**What is the significance of a spike or sharp wave on EEG?**

Signature of a potentially epileptogenic area in the region of brain originating the spike

**What is the most common EEG finding in complex partial seizures?**

Focal spikes, most commonly in the temporal region

**What percent of patients with complex partial seizures have a normal EEG?**

20–40%

**When is neuroimaging indicated in the evaluation of seizures?**

Evaluation of most types of partial seizures, especially when there is other evidence of neurologic dysfunction (e.g., hemiparesis) to suggest a symptomatic epilepsy
Seizures of adult onset if cause unknown

**What is the most sensitive and specific method to determine whether a spell is a seizure?**

Simultaneous video and EEG monitoring during a spell

**What EEG findings during a spell suggest pseudoseizure?**

Normal EEG

**Does lack of EEG change during a spell always exclude a seizure?**

No. Simple partial seizures (e.g., auras) are not usually accompanied by EEG changes.

## TREATMENT

**What is the generic name for each of the following brand name antiepileptic drugs (AEDs):**

- **Cerebyx**

  Fosphenytoin

- **Keppra**

  Levetiracetam

- **Dilantin**

  Phenytoin

- **Felbatol**

  Felbamate

- **Tegretol**

  Carbamazepine

- **Depakene**

  Valproic acid

- **Depakote**

  Divalproex sodium

- **Zarontin**

  Ethosuximide

- **Gabitril**

  Tiagabine

- **Mysoline**

  Primidone

- **Neurontin**              Gabapentin

- **Lamictal**               Lamotrigine

- **Topamax**                Topiramate

- **Trileptal**              Oxcarbazepine

- **Phenobarbital**          There is no common brand name

- **Zonegran**               Zonisamide

**What is the treatment of a provoked seizure?**

Relieving the provoking factor (e.g., correction of metabolic abnormalities)

**What is the treatment of a single seizure without an identifiable provoking factor?**

If the seizure is due to an epilepsy syndrome, then therapy may be initiated, depending on the natural history of the syndrome. If the etiology is unknown, then generally antiepileptic drugs are not initiated until after the second seizure, but this approach is controversial.

**Which AEDs are useful for simple and complex partial seizures as part of most epilepsy syndromes?**

All of them, except ethosuximide.

**What is the efficacy of these drugs for control of complex partial seizures in TLE?**

About 30% of patients continue to have complex partial seizures despite maximal drug therapy.

**What curative surgery is available for some patients with temporal lobe epilepsy?**

Resection of part of the temporal lobe–anterior temporal lobectomy

**How effective is it?**

70% become essentially seizure-free

**Which AED is useful only for absence seizures in childhood absence epilepsy?**

Ethosuximide

**How effective is it?**

It renders most patients with childhood absence epilepsy seizure free.

**What other AEDs are useful for absence seizures?**

The valproic acid derivatives, Depakote and Depakene

**Which AEDs are most useful for both myoclonic jerks and convulsions in JME?**

The valproic acid derivatives, Depakote and Depakene

**Which AEDs are the drugs of choice in patients with both partial and generalized seizures?**

The valproic acid derivatives, Depakote and Depakene

**What is the drug of choice for treatment of infantile spasms?**

Adrenocorticotropic hormone (ACTH) initially; valproic acid for maintenance therapy

**What is the most important factor determining the risk of seizure recurrence after withdrawal of AEDs?**

Etiology–the risk of seizure recurrence is determined by the natural history of the epilepsy syndrome. For example, patients with JME are well controlled with medications but almost universally have seizures when medication is withdrawn.

**What is the risk of seizure recurrence after medication withdrawal?**

20–70%, even for patients who are good candidates for drug withdrawal

# 9

# Dementia

**Give a five-word definition of dementia.**

Loss of previous intellectual ability

**What is a more comprehensive definition?**

Dementia is a clinical syndrome characterized by a significant decline in intellect from a previous higher level of functioning in an alert individual.

**What are four criteria for the diagnosis of dementia?**

1. Acquired memory impairment
2. Deficit of at least one other higher cortical function (e.g., judgement, praxis, language)
3. Impaired social or occupational functioning
4. Normal alertness (i.e., no delirium)

**How many causes are currently recognized?**

More than 75

**What is the most common cause?**

Alzheimer's disease, which accounts for approximately 50% of cases; also, in another 15%, Alzheimer's disease is present combined with a second disorder, such as vascular dementia or Parkinson's disease

**What is the second most common cause?**

Multiple cerebral infarcts, termed *multi-infarct dementia*

**Using the mnemonic VITAMIN, what are the treatable causes of dementia?**

**V**ascular: multiple strokes
**I**nfectious: neurosyphilis, chronic meningitis
**T**raumatic: subdural hematoma
**A**ffective: depression
**M**etabolic: hypothyroidism, chronic encephalopathies
**I**nflammatory: vasculitis, multiple sclerosis
**N**eoplasm or **N**ormal pressure hydrocephalus (NPH)

**In what percentage of dementia cases does a workup reveal a treatable cause?**

About 15%; 5% of patients have a reversible cause; in the other 10%, progression can be halted

**Describe a core laboratory workup for dementia.**

CT or MRI; CBC; ESR; blood chemistries, liver enzymes; thyroid function tests; $B_{12}$; syphilis serology Other tests may include CSF analysis, EEG, HIV testing, ANA, chest radiograph, EKG, or urinalysis

## ALZHEIMER'S DISEASE

**How is a definite diagnosis of Alzheimer's disease made?**

Autopsy or biopsy evidence of neuritic plaques and neurofibrillary tangles

**What are neuritic plaques?**

Small clumps of amorphous, silver-staining material scattered throughout the cerebral cortex, primarily composed of a core of amyloid surrounded by degenerated nerve processes and other material

**What are neurofibrillary tangles?**

Intraneuronal strands of silver-staining material

**Which neurotransmitter system is most affected?**

Acetylcholine, especially in the basal nucleus of Meynert

**What are the *clinical* criteria for probable Alzheimer's disease?**

1. Dementia demonstrated by exam and neuropsychological testing
2. Deficits in two or more cognitive areas
3. Progressive worsening of memory and other cognition
4. No disturbance of consciousness
5. Onset between ages 40 and 90
6. Patient has no other systemic disorder that causes dementia

**Are any curative treatments available for Alzheimer's disease?**

No, but cholinesterase inhibitors may improve cognition presumably by increasing cholinergic neurotransmission.

## MULTI-INFARCT DEMENTIA

**What is it?**

It is dementia resulting from more than one ischemic infarction, with or without other associated neurologic deficits.

**What is the association between the volume of infarcted brain and the severity of the dementia?**

The greater the extent of infarcted brain, the greater the dementia

**When associated with a major neurologic deficit, such as hemiparesis, is this dementia usually due to large or small vessel occlusion?**

Large vessel occlusion

**When occurring without other deficits, is this dementia usually due to large or small vessel occlusions?**

Small vessel occlusions

**What is another name for the small infarcts caused by small artery occlusion?**

Lacunes

**Where are lacunar infarcts frequently located?**

Scattered throughout subcortical grey and white matter

**What systemic disease predisposes a patient to these infarcts and thus to multi-infarct dementia?**

Untreated hypertension

**What is the eponym for lacunar infarcts scattered through cerebral white matter?**

Binswanger's disease

## NPH

**What is hydrocephalus?**

Dilated ventricles

**What are three causes of hydrocephalus?**

Obstructed CSF flow, decreased CSF absorption or, rarely, excessive production

**What is NPH?**

Ventricular dilatation with normal CSF pressure

**What is the postulated pathophysiology of NPH?**

Increased resistance to CSF absorption across the arachnoid villi

**How does ventricular dilation occur without increased intracranial pressure?**

Uncertain. Initially, impaired CSF absorption causes ventricles to swell and compact brain parenchyma; subsequently CSF production and absorption reach a new equilibrium and pressure returns to normal.

**What conditions may predispose patients to the development of NPH?**

Prior subarachnoid hemorrhage, head trauma, infection, Paget's disease; presumably, these act by obstructing CSF absorption by the arachnoid villi

**What percentage of patients with NPH have no predisposing condition?**

>50%

**What age group is typically affected by NPH?**

It rarely occurs before 60 years of age.

**What is the usual rate of onset?**

Subacute—develops over weeks, months, or years

**What is the classic triad of symptoms?**

Dementia, gait disturbance, and urinary incontinence

**What is the most common initial symptom?**

Gait disturbance

**What is the classic description of the gait disturbance associated with NPH?**

Magnetic gait (i.e., slow velocity; short, small steps), as though the feet are stuck to the floor

**What is the pathophysiology of incontinence associated with NPH?**

Dysfunction of subcortical fibers from frontal lobe to bladder control area of pons and cord, caused by pressure from expanding ventricles

**What is the CSF pressure in a normal person?**

80–180 mm water

| | |
|---|---|
| **What is the CSF opening pressure in a person with NPH?** | Normal |
| **What are the CT and MRI findings in NPH?** | Enlarged ventricles and periventricular hypodensity from subependymal CSF absorption |
| **What is hydrocephalus ex vacuo?** | Ventriculomegaly secondary to diffuse atrophy; it is distinguished from NPH by loss of brain parenchyma with a prominent sulcal pattern |
| **How is the diagnosis of NPH established?** | Temporary improvement of gait after removal of 30–50 ml of CSF from the lumbar subarachnoid space or by cisternography |
| **How long do the effects of a lumbar puncture last in a patient with NPH?** | Approximately 24 hours |
| **What are the long-term treatment options?** | Ventriculoperitoneal (or ventriculoatrial) shunt |
| **What is the prognosis of NPH?** | Approximately 50% of patients show improvement of symptoms after shunting; gait improves more than dementia |

## DEMENTIA WITH LEWY BODIES

| | |
|---|---|
| **When should you clinically suspect it?** | Rapidly progressing dementia and visual hallucinations |
| **Compare the Lewy bodies to Parkinson's disease.** | There are many more Lewy bodies present throughout the cortex and fewer in basal ganglia than in Parkinson's. |
| **What are Lewy bodies?** | Intracytoplasmic aggregates of alpha-synuclein (a protein) |

# 10  Sleep Disorders

| | |
|---|---|
| **What is the most common sleep disorder?** | Insomnia |
| **What is the daytime consequence of either narcolepsy or obstructive sleep apnea?** | Daytime sleepiness |
| **On average, how many hours does a healthy young American adult sleep?** | Six or seven |
| **What is the typical effect of depression on nocturnal sleep?** | Early awakening |
| **How is REM sleep clinically distinguished from non-REM sleep?** | REM is characterized by<br>1. Bursts of rapid eye movements<br>2. Accompanying hypotonia<br>3. Frequent dreaming |
| **How soon after sleep onset does REM sleep normally commence?** | Typically between 60 and 100 minutes |
| **Can REM episodes occur more than once during the night?** | Yes |

## NARCOLEPSY

| | |
|---|---|
| **What is the narcolepsy tetrad?** | Irresistible daytime sleepiness, cataplexy, hypnogogic hallucinations, sleep paralysis |
| **What is cataplexy?** | Sudden loss of muscle tone, especially after a strong emotional stimulus |
| **What is a hypnogogic hallucination?** | A vivid nocturnal dream-state hallucination |

| | |
|---|---|
| **What is sleep paralysis?** | Paralysis on awakening |
| **Characterize the sleep EEG in a person with narcolepsy.** | Early onset rapid eye movement (REM) sleep |
| **What is a multiple sleep latency test (MSLT)?** | A daytime test of sleepiness; EEG is monitored during four or five 20-minute naps every 2 hours in the EEG or sleep lab |
| **What MSLT result favors the diagnosis of narcolepsy?** | REM occurring at the beginning of sleep; "sleep-onset REM" |
| **What class of drugs ameliorates the daytime sleepiness?** | Stimulants, such as methylphenidate (Ritalin), dextroamphetamine, or modafinil (Provigil) |
| **What two classes of drugs ameliorate the cataplexy?** | Tricyclics, such as imipramine and GHB, gamma hydroxybutyrate (Xyrem) |

## OBSTRUCTIVE SLEEP APNEA

| | |
|---|---|
| **What happens to air flow during an episode of obstructive sleep apnea?** | It ceases |
| **Why?** | The pharynx becomes blocked |
| **What duration is abnormal?** | Ten seconds or more |
| **How is obstructive sleep apnea distinguished from central sleep apnea?** | Central: no abdominal and thoracic ventilatory effort<br>Obstructive: thoracic and abdominal efforts are present |
| **What is the usual body habitus in patients with obstructive sleep apnea?** | 75% are obese; 25% are normal weight. |
| **Characterize parapharyngeal fat in obstructive sleep apnea.** | Increased |

| | |
|---|---|
| **Characterize size of the oropharynx in obstructive sleep apnea.** | Decreased |
| **Name four treatment strategies for managing obstructive sleep apnea.** | 1. Weight loss<br>2. Nasal continuous positive airway pressure (CPAP)<br>3. Tracheostomy with daytime plugging<br>4. Avoidance of sedatives/alcohol |
| **What are three features of sleep in patients with obstructive sleep apnea?** | 1. Episodic apneas<br>2. Heroic snoring<br>3. Frequent awakening |

## NIGHTMARES AND NIGHT TERRORS

| | |
|---|---|
| **In what stage of sleep do nightmares occur?** | Usually REM sleep |
| **In what stage of sleep do night terrors occur?** | Usually stage 3 or 4 of non-REM sleep |
| **How long do they last?** | Several minutes to 1 hour |
| **Is treatment necessary?** | Seldom, with a benzodiazepine |
| **What clinically distinguishes a night terror from a nightmare?** | A night terror is characterized by brief, wild behavior; autonomic signs (tachycardia); and amnesia for the event. It occurs mostly in children.<br>A nightmare is simply a "bad dream," which the individual typically remembers after awakening. It occurs in both adults and children. |
| **What other sleep abnormality often accompanies night terrors?** | Sleep walking, or somnambulism |
| **Is any treatment necessary for night terrors?** | No |

## RESTLESS LEG SYNDROME AND PERIODIC LIMB MOVEMENTS

| | |
|---|---|
| **What is restless leg syndrome?** | Unpleasant leg sensations relieved by movement |

| | |
|---|---|
| **What time of day?** | Evening and night |
| **What is cause?** | Unknown |
| **What is treatment?** | Dopaminergic agonists |
| **What are periodic limb movements?** | Recurrent movements without the unpleasant sensations |
| **What is nocturnal myoclonus or sleep starts?** | Vigorous jerks at sleep onset, which do not recur |

## PARKINSON'S DISEASE AND ALLIED DISORDERS
### (See also Chapter 4)

| | |
|---|---|
| **What are the diagnostic pathologic findings of Parkinson's disease?** | Loss of pigmented nuclei in the substantia nigra with the presence of Lewy bodies |
| **What is the neurobiologic consequence?** | Depletion of dopamine in the striatum |
| **What is the striatum?** | Caudate nucleus and putamen of basal ganglia |
| **What is the common age of onset of Parkinson's disease?** | 40–70 years of age, with the peak incidence in the sixth decade |
| **What is the incidence of Parkinson's disease?** | Approximately 1% of the population over 50 years of age |
| **What are the three cardinal features of Parkinson's disease?** | Rest tremor, cogwheel rigidity, and bradykinesia |
| **What are eight additional signs caused by these features?** | Masked facies, loss of postural reflexes, decreased blink rate, small-stepped gait, hypovolemic voice, micrographia, gait arrest, backward falling |
| **Which cardinal feature is most specific for Parkinson's disease?** | Rest tremor |
| **Describe it.** | 3–5 Hz pill-rolling oscillation of the thumb and fingers at rest or when walking |
| **Describe the characteristic gait of Parkinson's disease?** | Short shuffling steps with a festinating, or hurried, quality. Gait initiation may be |

difficult and may be facilitated by having the patient step over an object.

**What diagnostic tests are necessary in the workup of Parkinson's disease?**

No diagnostic tests are necessary unless the patient is atypical.

**List six drugs that are effective in the treatment of Parkinson's disease.**

1. Carbidopa/levodopa (Sinemet)
2. Amantadine (Symmetrel)
3. Pramipexole (Mirapex) and ropinirole (Requip)
4. Selegiline (Eldepryl; Deprenyl)
5. Entacapone (Comtan)
6. Trihexyphenidyl (Artane)

**What is the mechanism of action of each of these drugs?**

1. Carbidopa/levodopa provides L-dopa (dihydroxyphenylalanine) to CNS, where it is converted into dopamine. Carbidopa reduces systemic breakdown of levodopa, maximizing the percent of the oral dose that reaches the brain.
2. Amantadine is a glutamate receptor (NMDA) antagonist in CNS.
3. Pramipexole and ropinirole are CNS dopamine agonists
4. Selegiline is a MAOB inhibitor and, thus, reduces the breakdown of dopamine in the synaptic cleft.
5. Entacapone prolongs dopamine duration by inhibition of COMT (catechol-O-methyl transferase), a dopamine-metabolizing enzyme.
6. Trihexyphenidyl blocks muscarinic cholinergic receptors, restoring acetylcholine-dopamine balance.

**Why is L-dopa more useful than dopamine to treat Parkinson's disease?**

The blood-brain barrier is permeable to L-dopa but not to dopamine.

**Why is carbidopa used in combination with L-dopa?**

Carbidopa prevents conversion of L-dopa to dopamine in peripheral tissues by inhibiting peripheral dopamine dehydroxylase.

**What are some common side effects of L-dopa?**

Dyskinesias, nausea/vomiting, nightmares or vivid dreams, and psychosis

**What is the difference between Parkinson's disease and parkinsonism?**

Parkinson's disease is an idiopathic disorder with classic neuropathology and responsive to L-dopa treatment. Parkinsonism is a clinical syndrome of many similar findings that is less responsive to dopamine.

**Name four identifiable causes of parkinsonism.**

Neuroleptic drug exposure; cerebrovascular disease; MPTP (methyl-phenyl-tetrahydropyridine); encephalitis lethargica (von Economo's disease)

**What is "parkinsonism plus?"**

Parkinson's manifestations plus other features not found in Parkinson's disease

**Name two movement disorders included in "parkinsonism plus."**

1. Progressive supranucler palsy (PSP)
2. Multiple System Atrophy

**What neurologic sign distinguishes PSP from Parkinson's disease?**

The PSP patient cannot look down.

**Name three multiple system atrophies.**

1. Striatonigral degeneration
2. Olivopontocerebellar atrophy
3. Primary autonomic insufficiency or Shy-Drager disease

**When is the term Shy-Drager appropriate?**

When orthostatic hypotension or other autonomic features predominate

**What class of disorders are "parkinsonism plus?"**

Degenerations of many neuronal systems including dopaminergic

**Are their causes known?**

No

## WILSON'S DISEASE (WD)

**What is hepatolenticular degeneration?**

Wilson's disease (WD)—a defect in copper metabolism that results in organ damage

**What organ systems are affected in WD?**

Liver, cornea, central nervous system, kidneys and reproductive system

**How common is WD?**

Uncommon; 1:30,000

**What is the minimum age of symptomatic onset?**

The onset of neurologic symptoms is usually after 6 years of age

**What is the mode of inheritance of WD?**

Autosomal recessive

**What chromosome carries the gene defect associated with WD?**

Chromosome 1

**What are four types of hepatic disease found in WD?**

Acute hepatitis, fulminant hepatic failure, chronic active hepatitis, cirrhosis

**What are the typical psychiatric manifestations of WD?**

Psychosis, personality changes, dementia

**What is the most common initial neurologic symptom of WD?**

Tremor

**What is a "wing-beating" tremor?**

A coarse tremor present, especially when the limbs are outstretched; it is a classic feature in WD

**What are the signs of severe WD and the areas of brain involvement?**

Basal ganglia dysfunction causes tremor, rigidity, chorea, and dystonia
Cortical dysfunction causes UMN signs.
Brain stem dysfunction causes dysarthria, drooling, dysphagia, and a "vacuous smile."
Cerebellar dysfunction causes ataxia.

**What is the pathognomonic ocular finding in WD?**

Kayser-Fleischer rings—golden ring of copper deposits in Descemet's membrane of the cornea

**What percentage of untreated WD patients with neurologic symptoms have Kayser-Fleischer rings?**

100%, eventually

**What ophthalmologic procedure helps visualize Kayser-Fleischer rings?**

A slit-lamp examination

| | |
|---|---|
| **What three laboratory tests confirm the diagnosis?** | 1. Low serum ceruloplasmin ($< 20$ mg/dl)<br>2. Elevated urinary excretion of copper ($> 100$ $\mu$g in 24 hours)<br>3. Increased concentration of copper in liver biopsy ($> 250$ $\mu$g/g dry weight) |
| **What are the typical MRI findings in WD?** | Increased signal and atrophy of the putamen, caudate, midbrain, pons, subcortical white matter, and cerebellum |
| **What are the findings on cerebral pathology in patients with WD?** | Nerve cell loss, especially in the basal ganglia; Alzheimer's type II astrocytes |
| **What is the medical treatment for WD?** | Penicillamine (or other chelator) |
| **What are possible side effects of medical therapy?** | Transient worsening of WD symptoms, rash, fever, leukopenia, thrombocytopenia, lymphadenopathy or proteinuria |
| **How long is medical therapy indicated?** | Life-long therapy is required |

## HUNTINGTON'S DISEASE

| | |
|---|---|
| **What type of disorder is it?** | Neurodegenerative |
| **Characterize a neurodegenerative disorder.** | Progressive death of a population of related neurons |
| **Name three other neurodegenerative disorders.** | Parkinson's disease, Alzheimer's disease, ALS |
| **What are the three cardinal clinical manifestations of Huntington's disease?** | Dementia, movement disorder, psychologic/psychiatric problems |
| **Characterize the movements.** | Chorea, athetosis, tremor |
| **What is a common eye movement abnormality?** | Impairment of saccades with preservation of smooth pursuits; patients usually blink to break fixation during saccadic testing |

| | |
|---|---|
| **What is the inheritance pattern?** | Autosomal dominant |
| **What is the penetrance?** | Complete |
| **What is its chromosomal location?** | Chromosome 4p |
| **What is the molecular genetic basis of Huntington's disease?** | Expansion of the number of repeats of the trinucleotide sequence CAG |
| **What are the three nucleotides of importance in Huntington's disease?** | Cytosine, adenine, and guanine |
| **What does the CAG sequence encode?** | The amino acid glutamine |
| **Correlate the length of the trinucleotide repeat with age of clinical onset.** | In general, the longer the sequence of trinucleotide repeats, the earlier the age of clinical onset |
| **What is anticipation?** | Succeeding generations experience earlier clinical onset and more severe disease. |
| **What is the molecular basis of anticipation?** | The trinucleotide repeat region is unstable and can expand further during replication, increasing the absolute number of trinucleotide repeats in the resultant cells. |
| **In Huntington's disease, is this more likely to occur during oogenesis or spermatogenesis?** | Spermatogenesis–therefore, anticipation is more likely to occur when Huntington's is inherited from the father |
| **What genetic analysis aids diagnosis in both symptomatic and presymptomatic persons?** | Molecular genetic testing to determine the number of trinucleotide repeats |
| **Why is presymptomatic diagnosis a weighty ethical issue?** | Huntington's disease may be diagnosed before symptoms appear, and this knowledge may prematurely affect the patient's quality of life. |

| | |
|---|---|
| Localize the major site of brain degeneration (neuronal loss). | Striatum |
| What is in the striatum and where is it? | Caudate nucleus and putamen in the basal ganglia |
| Name another area with significant neuronal loss. | Widely throughout the cerebral cortex |
| What is the typical age of clinical onset? | Thirties or forties |
| State the classic neuroimaging finding. | Atrophy of head of caudate with widening of lateral ventricles on MRI/CT |
| State three neuropsychiatric features. | Personality changes; dementia; psychosis or depression |
| What is the Westphal variant? | Akinetic rigidity, most common in juvenile onset |
| From which parent does the Westphal variant usually come? | The father |
| In Huntington's disease, what drugs are useful for symptomatic management? | |
| For chorea? | Haloperidol |
| For depression? | Tricyclics |
| For psychosis? | Neuroleptics |
| For anxiety? | Benzodiazepines |

## TOURETTE'S SYNDROME

| | |
|---|---|
| What is it? | Multiple motor and vocal tics |
| What is the typical age of onset? | 5–10 years of age |
| With what disorders is it associated? | Obsessive-compulsive disorder, attention deficit disorder |

| | |
|---|---|
| **What is the inheritance pattern?** | Autosomal dominant with reduced penetrance (probably on chromosome 18) |
| **What is a tic?** | It is a brief, stereotyped, repetitive movement of a body part. It may be semivolitional and associated with relief of tension. A tic can be mimicked. |
| **How are tics classified?** | Simple: isolated movement of a body part (e.g., shoulder shrug, eyelid blinking, head rolling)<br>Complex: semipurposeful movements (e.g., jumping, touching)<br>Vocal: brief outbursts of speech or sounds |
| **What feature of the vocal tics may be characteristic of Tourette's syndrome?** | Coprolalia (i.e., obscenity), echolalia (i.e., repetition of a phrase), profanity |
| **Is coprolalia a common feature?** | No |
| **How is Tourette's treated?** | Neuroleptics, especially haloperidol (Haldol) and pimozide (Orap), help reduce tics. Clonidine, an alpha agonist, may also reduce tics. |

## DYSTONIA

### IDIOPATHIC TORSION DYSTONIA

| | |
|---|---|
| **What is dystonia?** | An involuntary sustained contraction of agonist and antagonist muscles, usually causing repetitive, twisting movements or abnormal postures |
| **What is blepharospasm?** | Involuntary forced eye closure |
| **What is torticollis?** | Involuntary sustained contractions of the cervical musculature, resulting in pain and abnormal head positioning |
| **What is writer's cramp?** | A type of dystonia that is brought on by a particular action (in this case, writing) |
| **What is spasmodic dysphonia?** | Strangled speech due to spasm of phonatory muscles |

**What is Meige syndrome?**

Blepharospasm and oromandibular dystonia

**What are two systemic drug treatments for dystonia?**

Anticholinergic drugs and benzodiazepines are useful.

**How does botulinum A toxin work?**

Botox is injected directly into affected muscles and inhibits release of acetylcholine at the neuromuscular junction, partially paralyzing the affected muscles. It takes about 1 week to reach maximal effect and usually lasts for a few months.

**What is an important acute cause of dystonia, especially torticollis?**

Neuroleptic agents (e.g., antipsychotics, antiemetics), especially in children

# 12

# Spine and Spinal Cord Disorders

## CORD SYNDROMES

**Occlusion of what blood vessel is the most common cause of a vascular spinal cord syndrome?**

The anterior spinal artery

**What is the name of the anatomic syndrome caused by this occlusion?**

Anterior cord syndrome

**What three sensations are spared in the anterior cord syndrome?**

Vibration, position, deep pain (posterior column functions)

**What pathways are injured in this syndrome?**

Corticospinal (motor) and lateral spinothalamic (pain/temperature) tracts

**What are the most important tracts affected in a *posterior cord syndrome?***

The dorsal columns (also called the posterior columns)

**What are the manifestations of dorsal column injury?**

Loss of position, deep pain, and vibration sensibility below the lesion out of proportion to motor deficit. Paresthesias may also occur.

**What is the cardinal neurologic finding of a *central cord syndrome?***

A transverse band (girdle) across the body in which pain and temperature perception are lost

**What is another name for this?**

A dissociated, suspended sensory loss

**Why does sensory loss occur in this distribution?**

Corticospinal, posterior column, *and* lateral spinothalamic tracts are spared. Only segmental pain and temperature fibers are disrupted as they cross the midline to enter the contralateral ascending lateral spinothalamic tracts.

**If the central lesion expands, what are the motor consequences?**

LMN signs at the affected segment because of extension into the anterior horns

UMN signs below the lesion because of corticospinal tract involvement

**What is the classic cause of a central cord syndrome?**

Syringomyelia

**What are two traumatic causes?**

Traumatic syrinx and central cord hemorrhage

**What is the eponym for a syndrome caused by hemisection of the spinal cord?**

Brown-Séquard syndrome

**What are its manifestations?**

1. Ipsilateral corticospinal tract damage (UMN paralysis)
2. Ipsilateral loss of posterior column function (position and vibration)
3. *Contralateral* loss of spinothalamic function (pain and temperature)
4. Light touch unaffected

**What is its most common cause?**

Tumor

**At what vertebral level does the spinal cord end in adults?**

About L1

**What is the cauda equina?**

Gathered roots of L2 and below; they occupy the spinal canal below the cord

**What is the conus medullaris?**

The bottom tip of the cord

**Choosing between a cauda equina and conus medullaris syndrome:**
**Which is likely to cause asymmetric leg LMN signs?**

Cauda equina syndrome

| | |
|---|---|
| **Which is likely to cause asymmetric leg dermatomal sensory deficits?** | Cauda equina syndrome |
| **Which is likely to cause bowel or bladder incontinence, and why?** | Conus medullaris syndrome—the conus medullaris is at the most inferior extent of the spinal cord where a lesion primarily affects sacral roots to the bowel and bladder |

## ACUTE CORD INJURIES

| | |
|---|---|
| **Why is acute spinal cord compression an emergency?** | Because treatment within 6 hours of onset may permit good outcome |
| **What are three physical exam findings of spinal shock?** | Paralysis with areflexia<br>Sensory loss<br>Autonomic paralysis<br>All three occur below the level of the lesion |
| **What is the etiology of spinal shock?** | Acute cord injury |
| **What spinal cord region is most frequently injured?** | Cervical |
| **Name two life-threatening complications of acute high cervical cord injury.** | 1. Inability to breathe: loss of phrenic (C3, C4) and intercostal nerve function<br>2. Hypotension: autonomic dysfunction |
| **What is the characteristic sensory consequence of a cervical or thoracic cord injury?** | Bilateral sensory loss below the lesion (e.g., the legs, trunk, or applicable areas of upper extremity) |
| **What is this type of sensory deficit called?** | A "sensory level" deficit |
| **What is the motor deficit of cervical cord injury?** | Tetraplegia (quadriplegia) |

| | |
|---|---|
| **What are five common medical complications of quadriplegia?** | Pneumonia, deep vein thrombosis with pulmonary embolization, decubitus ulcers, urinary retention, and bladder infections |
| **What test is used to determine if the cord is anatomically disrupted?** | MRI |
| **What are five steps in early management of high cervical cord trauma?** | 1. ABCs of resuscitation (i.e., airway, breathing, circulation) 2. Immobilization 3. Nasogastric feeding tube 4. Urinary catheterization 5. Venous access and high dose IV steroids |
| **Is methyl prednisolone useful in acute spinal cord injury?** | Yes |

## SPINAL STENOSIS

| | |
|---|---|
| **What is it?** | Narrowing of the diameter of the spinal canal |
| **What spinal levels are most commonly involved?** | Mid-to-lower cervical and lumbar levels |
| **Who is at risk for symptomatic spinal stenosis?** | 1. Patients with severe, congenital spinal stenosis (e.g., achondroplastic dwarfs) 2. Patients with mild congenital narrowed canals and superimposed bony degeneration or disc herniation 3. Patients who have previously undergone extensive spinal surgery |
| **What are the potential neurologic consequences of spinal stenosis?** | Compression of the spinal cord, spinal roots, or surrounding vascular structures; this may cause compressive or ischemic cord symptoms (e.g., myelopathy) or spinal root symptoms (e.g., radiculopathy) |
| **What are the symptoms of significant cervical stenosis?** | Neck stiffness, pain and numbness in the neck and shoulders that may radiate into one or both arms, weakness in one or both arms, gait impairment |

**What are the signs of significant cervical stenosis on exam?**

Limited range of neck motion, dermatomal sensory loss in one or both arms, LMN signs in one or both arms, and UMN signs in one or both legs

**What is Lhermitte's sign?**

The production of a shock-like sensation radiating down the spine when the neck is flexed; it is caused by conditions that affect the posterior columns

**What increases the likelihood that cervical stenosis will be symptomatic?**

Extreme neck rotation (e.g., when backing up an automobile)
Muscle relaxation during sleep, especially on the "wrong" pillow
Whiplash injuries

**What are the symptoms of significant lumbar stenosis?**

Low back, hip, and buttock pain that may extend into one or both legs and is sometimes accompanied by leg weakness; disturbances in bowel, bladder, and erectile function may also be seen

**What precipitates these symptoms?**

Standing, walking, or extension at the waist

**What relieves these symptoms?**

Sitting, lying down, or flexing the waist

**What are the signs of significant lumbar stenosis on exam?**

Flexed posture at the waist, dermatomal sensory loss in one or both legs, and LMN signs in one or both legs

**What is neurogenic claudication?**

Precipitation of symptoms of lumbar stenosis during ambulation, presumably because of ischemia of lumbosacral roots

**What is spondylosis?**

Degenerative spinal osteoarthritis, which may narrow the spinal canal or neuroforamina

**What is spondylolisthesis?**

Anterior subluxation of one vertebral body over another

**At what spinal levels is spondylolisthesis usually seen?**

L5 on S1
L4 on L5

**What are the potential neurologic consequences of spondylolisthesis?**

Compression of nerve roots or spinal cord due to spinal stenosis

**What four pathologic conditions should be considered in the differential diagnosis of potential spinal stenosis?**

1. Large, central herniated nucleus pulposus (HNP) with resultant cord or nerve root compression
2. Intra- or extra-medullary mass lesion, such as tumor or abscess
3. Demyelinating lesion of the cord
4. Spinal cord infarct

Cervical stenosis may also mimic the UMN and LMN signs of ALS.

**Are plain radiographs useful in the evaluation of spinal stenosis?**

Yes, because the degree of bony narrowing is seen better than it is on MRI

**What additional imaging studies may be helpful?**

CT-myelogram and MRI provide more detailed information about soft tissue, such as spinal cord and roots, than do plain radiographs

**What electrophysiologic studies may be helpful?**

Electromyogram (EMG) and nerve conduction studies (NCS) may demonstrate evidence of active denervation caused by myelopathy or radiculopathy. Somatosensory evoked potentials (SSEP) may help localize the level of dysfunction, if sensory symptoms are present.

**What is the typical course of therapy for symptomatic cervical stenosis?**

NSAIDs, muscle relaxants, cervical collar, traction, and physical therapy

**For symptomatic lumbar stenosis?**

NSAIDs, muscle relaxants, and rest, followed by physical therapy

**When is surgery indicated?**

When symptoms fail to respond to conservative therapy or if deficits progress despite conservative therapy

## HNP (HERNIATED DISC)

**What is the nucleus pulposus?**

The gel-like center within the annulus fibrosis of an intervertebral disc

**What is HNP?**

Extrusion of this gel-like material through the annulus, usually in a posterolateral direction, due to annulus degeneration or trauma

**What is the typical neurologic consequence of an HNP?**

Compression of an exiting spinal nerve root, resulting in a radiculopathy

**Which lumbar discs are most susceptible to herniation?**

L5–S1, then L4–L5

**Which lumbar roots are most often affected?**

S1 and L5

**Why?**

Because **lumbar** discs usually compress the root exiting one interspace below that of the affected disc

**Which cervical discs are most susceptible to herniation?**

C6–C7, then C5–C6

**Which cervical roots are most often affected?**

C7 and C6

**Why?**

Because **cervical** discs usually compress the root exiting at the same interspace as the affected disc

**How can you remember these relationships?**

The *affected root's number* corresponds to the second number of the herniating disc. This means that an L4–L5 disc compresses the L5 nerve root, even though L5 exits below the L5 vertebra.

**Why is the relation between a herniated disc and affected nerve root so complicated?**

1. There are seven cervical vertebrae and eight cervical nerves, so C7 exits *above* and C8 exits *below* vertebra C7.
2. The anatomic relationship between a herniating disc and an emerging nerve root differs between cervical and lumbar discs. Lumbosacral discs compress the nerve root that emerges one interspace below the disc, but cervical discs compress the root at the same level as the disc.

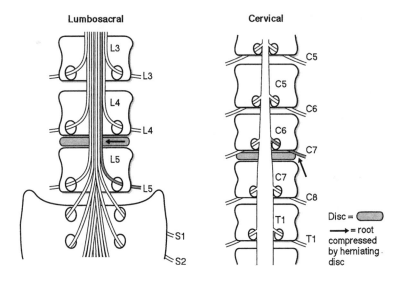

| | |
|---|---|
| **What are the symptoms of lumbar or cervical radiculopathy?** | Low back or neck pain that radiates into an extremity in the distribution of a particular nerve root<br>Tingling in a particular dermatome or weakness of muscles innervated by a particular nerve root |
| **Why is radiculopathic pain worsened by coughing, sneezing, or straining at stool?** | Increased CSF pressure shifts nerve roots |
| **What is sciatica?** | It is pain that radiates down the posterior aspect of the leg in the distribution of the sciatic nerve. It is most often due to HNP affecting L4, L5, or S1. |
| **What are the signs of radiculopathy on neurologic exam?** | Atrophy, hypotonia, and weakness of muscles innervated by a particular nerve root<br>Absent or hypoactive deep tendon reflex corresponding to a particular nerve root<br>Sensory abnormalities in a particular dermatome |

Correlate weakness,
decreased reflexes, and
sensory changes with C5,
C6, L5, and S1
radiculopathies.

**Table 12–1.    Characteristics of Radiculopathies**

| Radiculopathy at: | Weakness | Hyporeflexia | Sensory Changes |
|---|---|---|---|
| C5 | Deltoid muscle | Biceps | Patch on shoulder |
| C6 | Biceps muscle | Biceps | Thumb side of hand |
| L5 | Foot, first toe dorsiflexion | *** | Dorsum of foot; lateral ankle; first toe |
| S1 | Foot plantar flexion | Ankle | Posterolateral calf; fifth toe |

| | |
|---|---|
| **What is Lasègue's sign? or "straight leg raising sign"?** | In the supine position, a patient feels back pain that radiates into the leg when the leg is flexed at the hip and then extended at the knee. This suggests an L4, L5, or S1 radiculopathy. |
| **What is Spurling's sign?** | The production of pain radiating into the arm when downward pressure is placed on the head with the head tilted towards the symptomatic side; its presence is suggestive of a cervical radiculopathy |
| **What findings may be present on plain radiographs of a lumbar or cervical HNP?** | Disc space narrowing at the corresponding level |
| **What other imaging studies are more useful in the evaluation of a potential HNP?** | Spinal MRI and CT-myelogram |
| **What is a Schmorl's nodule?** | The radiographic appearance of a disc that has herniated into the adjacent vertebral body |

| | |
|---|---|
| **What electrophysiologic studies may be helpful in the evaluation of possible radiculopathy?** | EMG and NCS |
| **What is the preferred course of therapy for a symptomatic HNP?** | The vast majority of patients recover with NSAIDs and avoidance of provocative activities. Some physicians advocate muscle relaxants, bed rest, physical therapy, exercise, and weight loss. |
| **When is surgery indicated?** | If symptoms fail to respond to conservative measures or if there is intractable pain, continuing weakness, or signs of cord or cauda equina compression (e.g., incontinence) |
| **What direction of disc herniation would cause cord compression?** | Central herniation |
| **What are the common approaches to surgical intervention?** | The typical procedure is a hemilaminectomy and discectomy with or without foraminotomy or vertebral body fusion; the approach is posterior in the lumbar region but may be anterior or posterior in the cervical region. |
| **What are some common causes of recurrent symptoms after surgical intervention?** | Radiculopathy due to residual disc material, scar tissue, or recurrent HNP at the same or different level |
| **What may contribute to poor outcome and continuing pain?** | Inactivity and obesity |

## MYELITIS

| | |
|---|---|
| **What distinguishes myelitis from myelopathy?** | In myelitis, there is spinal cord inflammation, which is one cause of myelopathy. |
| **What defines a transverse myelitis?** | Bilateral cord involvement |
| **Which cord pathways are involved?** | All of them |

## Spinal Cord Anatomy

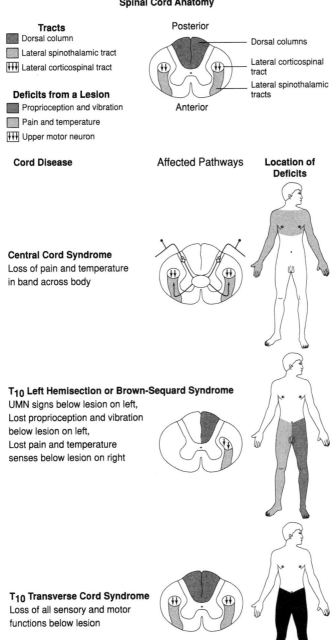

**Tracts**
- ▨ Dorsal column
- ▨ Lateral spinothalamic tract
- ⊞ Lateral corticospinal tract

**Deficits from a Lesion**
- ▨ Proprioception and vibration
- ▨ Pain and temperature
- ⊞ Upper motor neuron

Posterior

Dorsal columns

Lateral corticospinal tract

Lateral spinothalamic tracts

Anterior

**Cord Disease**  **Affected Pathways**  **Location of Deficits**

**Central Cord Syndrome**
Loss of pain and temperature
in band across body

**T₁₀ Left Hemisection or Brown-Sequard Syndrome**
UMN signs below lesion on left,
Lost proprioception and vibration
below lesion on left,
Lost pain and temperature
senses below lesion on right

**T₁₀ Transverse Cord Syndrome**
Loss of all sensory and motor
functions below lesion

| | |
|---|---|
| **Is transverse myelitis a syndrome or a diagnosis?** | Syndrome |
| **What are the three recognized causes?** | Postinfectious, postvaccinial, and multiple sclerosis |
| **What is the presumed common thread among these etiologies?** | It is presumably immunologic in origin. |
| **What are three microscopic findings of myelitis?** | Necrosis, inflammation, and demyelination |
| **What is the typical course of myelitis?** | Onset of back pain, followed by weakness and paralysis below the involved cord level |
| **Is it usually monophasic or multiphasic?** | Monophasic |
| **What is the usual diagnosis when multiphasic?** | Multiple sclerosis |
| **What eponym applies to optic neuritis and transverse myelitis?** | Devic's syndrome |
| **Describe urinary function in a person with transverse myelitis.** | Acute retention followed by overflow incontinence |
| **What are the CSF changes?** | There is often an increase in lymphocytes. |
| **What abnormalities may imaging studies show?** | Questionable swelling of a few contiguous cord segments; MRI may show increased T2 signal intensity |
| **What do SSEPs show?** | Slowed central conduction time or absence of a scalp response to stimulation of a peripheral nerve |
| **What are typical deep tendon reflex findings?** | Acute: absent (spinal shock)<br>Chronic: hyperactive with Babinski's sign and ankle clonus |

## TUMORS AND CHRONIC CORD COMPRESSION

| | |
|---|---|
| **What are the signs and symptoms of spinal cord compression?** | Back or radicular pain at level of lesion<br>UMN weakness, sensory loss, and bladder dysfunction below the lesion |
| **What are seven non-tumor causes of chronic cord compression?** | HNP<br>Vertebral osteoarthritis (spondylosis)<br>Vertebral compression fracture<br>Vertebral dislocation<br>Hematoma<br>Abscess or granuloma<br>Foreign body (e.g., bullet) |
| **What are the radiographic studies of choice for imaging spinal cord compression?** | MRI and/or CT myelography |
| **What percent of primary CNS tumors arise in the spinal cord?** | About 15% |
| **Distinguish between an intramedullary and an extramedullary-intradural tumor.** | An intramedullary tumor is within the spinal cord parenchyma, whereas an extramedullary–intradural is inside the dura but not within the cord. |
| **Name two common extramedullary-intradural tumors.** | Meningioma and schwannoma (neurofibroma) |
| **Name three common intramedullary glial tumors.** | Astrocytoma, ependymoma, glioblastoma |
| **Where are most metastatic tumors located?** | Extradural space |
| **Metastatic involvement of the cord should be especially suspected in:** | Anyone with known primary neoplasm and new cord complaints including urinary difficulties |

| | |
|---|---|
| **What percentage of patients with spinal cord metastases will have two or more lesions?** | Approximately 15%–25% |
| **Name three treatment choices for metastatic cord tumors.** | IV corticosteroids, radiation, or surgical decompression |

## LOW BACK PAIN SYMPTOMOLOGY

| | |
|---|---|
| **Is most back pain neurologic or musculoskeletal in origin?** | Musculoskeletal |
| **Which distribution favors disc (nucleus pulposus) herniation?** | Unilateral, especially with extension into thigh or leg |
| **Which favors spinal stenosis?** | Walking-induced |
| **Which favors sacroiliac arthritis?** | Tenderness in sacroiliac dimple |
| **Which favors degenerative arthritis of vertebral facets?** | Worse after spine extension or prolonged sitting |
| **What are the facets?** | Where one vertebra opposes or rests upon another |
| **What imaging study best identifies H.N.P.?** | Axial spine MRI |

# 13

# Peripheral Nerve Disorders

## ANATOMY

**From what structure do the peripheral nerves of the upper extremity arise?**

The brachial plexus

**What nerves in the arm originate in the brachial plexus?**

Median, ulnar, radial, musculocutaneous, and axillary nerves

**Which of these nerves extend into the forearm?**

Radial, median, and ulnar nerves

**From which nerve roots is the brachial plexus formed?**

C5–T1

**What mnemonic is used to recall the five components of the brachial plexus?**

Republicans Think Democrats Can't Negotiate (**R**oots, **T**runks, **D**ivisions, **C**ords, and **N**erves)

On the following figure, trace the pathways of the C6 nerve root through the brachial plexus out to the median nerve, C7 out to the radial nerve, and C8 nerve root out to the ulnar nerve.

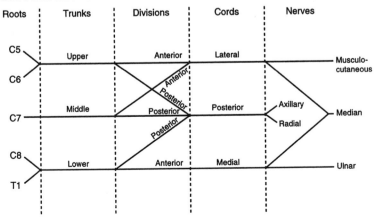

**The peripheral nerves of the lower extremity arise from what structure?**

The lumbosacral plexus

**The lumbosacral plexus arises from which nerve roots?**

L2–S2

**What is a plexus?**

A plexus takes roots and weaves them into peripheral nerves.

**The paraspinal muscles receive innervation via which ramus of a peripheral nerve?**

The dorsal rami of the cervical, thoracic, lumbar, and sacral spinal nerves

**Why is this important?**

The electromyographer uses EMG abnormalities in paraspinal muscles to help differentiate a radiculopathy (proximal) from a neuropathy (peripheral). Paraspinal muscle denervation suggests a lesion in the nerve root (i.e., radiculopathy).

**Spinal nerves are formed from which structures?**

The ventral and dorsal (motor and sensory) roots of all spinal cord segments except C1, which has no sensory root

**What is a dermatome?**

The area of skin supplied by a spinal nerve

**Does the dorsal root ganglion lie proximal or distal to the formation of a spinal nerve?**

Proximal

**What are the two major components of a peripheral nerve?**

The axon and myelin sheath

## PERIPHERAL NEUROPATHY

**Divide chronic and subacute peripheral neuropathies into two etiologic groups.**

Inherited and acquired

**What is the most common inherited neuropathy?**

Charcot-Marie-Tooth disease (hereditary motor-sensory neuropathy type I)

| | |
|---|---|
| **Name a hereditary predisposition to pressure palsy (compression neuropathy).** | Tomaculous neuropathy |
| **What are four common causes of acquired neuropathies?** | 1. Diabetes<br>2. Alcohol<br>3. Uremia<br>4. Drugs (e.g., chemotherapeutic agents) |
| **Can paraneoplastic disease produce peripheral neuropathy?** | Yes |
| **Does diabetes have to produce symptomatic hyperglycemia before peripheral neuropathy develops?** | No. Peripheral neuropathy may be the presenting complaint. |
| **What are some potential autonomic manifestations of peripheral neuropathy?** | Altered sweating, changes in skin color, orthostatic hypotension, constipation, impotence, and urinary incontinence |
| **What are two heavy metal causes of peripheral neuropathy.** | Lead and arsenic |
| **What are Mees' lines?** | Transverse white lines in the fingernails or toenails caused by arsenic poisoning |
| **List three common symptoms of peripheral neuropathy?** | Tingling, burning, and numbness—known as paresthesia, these abnormal spontaneous sensations are common in peripheral neuropathy |
| **What is the distribution of symptoms?** | The distal bilateral upper and lower extremities (so-called stocking-and-glove distribution) |
| **What are the physical findings of peripheral neuropathy?** | Muscle atrophy, weakness, sensory deficits and hyporeflexia in a predominantly distal distribution |
| **What abnormal movements might occur with a peripheral neuropathy?** | Fasciculation and pseudoathetosis |

**What are fasciculations?**

Visible twitches in a muscle caused by spontaneous discharges of motor units; looks like a bag of worms moving under the skin

**Are fasciculations always pathologic?**

No. Benign fasciculations are common in normal individuals after vigorous exercise, fatigue, dehydration, or excessive caffeine intake.

**What is pseudoathetosis?**

Writhing, snake-like movements caused by a loss of proprioception in the distal extremities that occur in severe peripheral neuropathy

**What four sensory modalities should be checked when assessing a peripheral neuropathy?**

Vibration, proprioception, light touch, pain (pin-prick), and temperature

**How is a clinically suspected peripheral neuropathy confirmed?**

Nerve conduction studies and EMG. (Use of the term EMG is, generally, assumed to refer to both.)

**What are three major classifications of peripheral neuropathy based on nerve conduction studies?**

Motor and sensory nerves may be affected individually or selectively within each classification:
1. Primary demyelinating
2. Primary axonal
3. Mixed demyelinating and axonal neuropathy

**What is the major electrophysiologic characteristic of a demyelinating neuropathy?**

Slowing of conduction velocity

**What are the major electrophysiologic characteristics of an axonal neuropathy?**

1. Decreased amplitude of the compound muscle/sensory action potential
2. Denervation in the affected muscles
3. Little or no slowing of conduction velocity

**Is there a direct correlation between the abnormalities found on EMG and clinical examination?**

No. There may be significant clinical findings with minimal electrophysiologic changes and vice versa.

**What are the indications for nerve biopsy?**

Although nerve biopsies are seldom needed, they are indicated when vasculitis or amyloidosis is suspected.

**Which nerve should be biopsied, and why?**

The sural nerve is chosen most frequently because injury to this nerve causes numbness in a very small area of the calf.

**For each pathologic finding, name some causative factors, conditions, or diseases:**

**Demyelination?**

Guillian-Barré syndrome, diabetes, uremia, Charcot-Marie-Tooth disease

**Axonal loss?**

Alcohol, diabetes, uremia, chemotherapy (e.g., vincristine)

**Amyloid deposition?**

Familial or acquired amyloidosis

**Focal myelin thickening?**

Tomaculous neuropathy

**Vasculitis?**

Polyarteritis nodosa and other connective tissue diseases
(**Note:** Most neuropathies have some overlap of pathologic findings, particularly demyelination and axonal loss.)

**What screening lab tests should be ordered when evaluating peripheral neuropathy?**

Serum glucose, BUN, creatinine, sedimentation rate, protein electrophoresis, antinuclear antibody, and rheumatoid factor; always consider HIV testing; anti-MAG, anti-GM2, and antineuronal antibodies are useful in some cases

**Name two peripheral neuropathies that can be diagnosed by genetic testing?**

Charcot-Marie-Tooth disease and tomaculous neuropathy

**A gene duplication is associated with which?**

Charcot-Marie-Tooth disease

**A gene deletion is associated with which?**

Tomaculous neuropathy

| | |
|---|---|
| **What are the common treatments for the sensory symptoms of peripheral neuropathies?** | Tricyclic antidepressants (e.g. amitriptyline), anticonvulsants (e.g. gabapentin), and topical agents (capsaicin) |

## MONONEURITIS MULTIPLEX

| | |
|---|---|
| **What is mononeuritis multiplex?** | A descriptive term for inflammation of several different nerves; the clinical presentation is usually subacute or chronic |
| **How does one determine which nerves are involved?** | The determination is based on which muscles are affected and the distribution of sensory deficits. |
| **What is the most common cause of mononeuritis multiplex?** | Vasculitic neuropathy (e.g., polyarteritis nodosa) |
| **How is vasculitic neuropathy confirmed?** | Nerve biopsy |
| **What is the most common treatment for mononeuritis multiplex?** | Immunosuppression with corticosteroids |

## COMPRESSION NEUROPATHY

| | |
|---|---|
| **What is a compression neuropathy?** | Focal nerve injury secondary to chronic trauma |
| **What is the most common compression neuropathy?** | Median neuropathy at the wrist (carpal tunnel syndrome) |
| **What are some other common compression neuropathies?** | Ulnar neuropathy at the elbow, radial neuropathy at the humerus (Saturday night palsy), and peroneal neuropathy at the fibular head |
| **Name two common causes of peroneal neuropathy.** | 1. Crossing of the legs<br>2. Improper positioning during surgery |
| **How are compression neuropathies diagnosed?** | Clinical and electrophysiologic evaluation |

| | |
|---|---|
| **What are the four intrinsic hand muscles supplied by the median nerve?** | LOAF muscles: **L**umbricals I and II; **O**pponens pollicis, **A**bductor pollicis brevis, **F**lexor pollicis brevis (superficial head) |
| **What is the characteristic NCV finding of a compression neuropathy?** | Focal slowing or conduction block at the point of compression |
| **What information does an EMG needle examination provide about a compression neuropathy?** | The presence of denervation, which suggests the severity of nerve injury and prognosis |
| **How are compression neuropathies treated?** | Relief of the compression, which can be accomplished by: 1. Stopping the precipitating activity 2. Prescribing anti-inflammatory medications 3. Splinting or padding the site of compression 4. Surgical decompression |

## GUILLAIN-BARRÉ SYNDROME

| | |
|---|---|
| **How does it usually present?** | Distal paresthesias followed by ascending weakness that begins in the legs and moves up to the arms progressively over several days |
| **What is the most common antecedent illness?** | *Campylobacter jejuni* gastroenteritis |
| **What are other common antecedent illnesses?** | Preceding viral illness, such as gastroenteritis or upper respiratory infections |
| **What time of year has the highest incidence?** | During the winter, probably because of increased viral gastroenteritis and respiratory infections |
| **What are key physical exam findings?** | Symmetrical proximal and distal weakness with areflexia; sensory loss is usually minimal |

**Distinguish the leg paresthesias of Guillain-Barré from those of transverse myelitis.**

Transverse myelitis causes paresthesias above the inguinal ligament area.

**What is the characteristic CSF finding?**

Elevated protein (>55 mg/dl) without a significant pleocytosis; "albuminocytological dissociation"

**What do nerve conduction studies show?**

Early: normal; possibly prolonged or absent F waves
Late: marked slowing with conduction block (and temporal dispersion of the wave form)

**What is the Miller-Fisher variant?**

Ophthalmoplegia (bulbar Guillain-Barré syndrome), ataxia, and areflexia

**What is the acute management of Guillain-Barré syndrome?**

Hospitalization, often in an ICU
Vital capacity must be frequently monitored.
Elective intubation with or without ventilatory support is indicated if vital capacity becomes <15 ml/kg (~1 liter in adults).

**What treatments modify disease course?**

Plasma exchange and I.V.I.G. reduces duration of disability.

**What is the prognosis?**

About 5% of patients die from complications that are largely avoidable. Most people become ambulatory again. A small minority (10%) may be permanently disabled.

**What is the course?**

Variable, recovery may take up to a year or more in a few patients

**What are three life-threatening complications?**

1. Upper airway obstruction due to pharyngeal muscle paralysis
2. Respiratory muscle failure
3. Autonomic dysfunction with cardiac arrhythmias or hypotension because of autonomic instability

## CHRONIC INFLAMMATORY DEMYELINATING PERIPHERAL NEUROPATHY (CIDP)

| | |
|---|---|
| **What is CIDP?** | A recurring form of peripheral neuropathy |
| **What is the pathogenesis?** | An acquired, inflammatory demyelination of peripheral nerves and nerve roots of unknown etiology |
| **What is evidence of an immune etiology?** | Mononuclear cell infiltration of peripheral nerve myelin indicates a defect of cellular immunity. Its responsiveness to plasma exchange implicates the humoral immune system. |
| **What are typical symptoms?** | Diffuse, symmetrical weakness with variable sensory complaints progressing and recurring over weeks to months |
| **What are the findings on examination?** | Weakness, depressed or absent deep tendon reflexes, and variable sensory deficits |
| **What is the distribution of weakness?** | Weakness usually is symmetric and proximal (rather than distal, as occurs in other peripheral neuropathies) |
| **What are CSF findings?** | Elevated protein without pleocytosis; "albuminocytological dissociation" |
| **What do nerve conduction studies show?** | Marked slowing of conduction velocity with "conduction block" |
| **What four conditions can mimic idiopathic CIDP?** | 1. Guillain-Barré syndrome 2. Lyme polyneuropathy 3. HIV-associated CIDP 4. Demyelinating neuropathies associated with monoclonal antibodies |
| **How does CIDP differ from Guillain-Barré syndrome?** | CIPD progresses for several months with frequent relapses, whereas Guillain-Barré is acute and monophasic. |

**What is the standard treatment?**

Immunosuppressive therapy—usually high-dose prednisone, although plasma exchange and intravenous gamma globulin are also used

**What is the prognosis of this condition?**

More than 90% of patients will respond to immunosuppressive drugs; however, the relapse rate is high, which often necessitates long-term treatment.

# 14

# Myasthenia Gravis and Other Neuromuscular Junction Disorders

## MYASTHENIA GRAVIS

| | |
|---|---|
| **What is myasthenia gravis?** | Weakness due to a defect of neuromuscular transmission |
| **What neurotransmitter is involved?** | Acetylcholine (ACh) |
| **Is the ACh nicotinic or muscarinic?** | Nicotinic |
| **What causes the defect in neuromuscular transmission?** | Autoantibodies directed against the nicotinic ACh receptor on skeletal muscle, usually against the binding site for ACh (alpha subunit) |
| **How does this affect the ACh receptor?** | It accelerates degradation of the ACh receptor and blocks the ACh-binding site. |
| **In the untreated patient, what three histopathologic changes are seen at the neuromuscular junction?** | 1. Simplification of the postsynaptic membrane<br>2. Widening of the synaptic cleft<br>3. Decreased number of ACh receptors |
| **What is the role of the thymus in the pathophysiology of myasthenia gravis?** | Thymic T cells probably augment B-cell production of autoantibodies |
| **Name three other autoimmune diseases associated with myasthenia gravis?** | Graves' disease, collagen-vascular diseases, pernicious anemia |

**What is the cardinal clinical manifestation of myasthenia gravis?**

Fatigable weakness of skeletal muscle

**Define *fatigable*.**

The patient's strength decreases with successive muscle contractions.

**What is the effect of a brief rest?**

The patient's strength improves.

**Which muscles are most frequently involved?**

Extraocular and eyelid muscles, resulting in fluctuating diplopia and ptosis

**What other muscles are commonly involved?**

Facial, oropharyngeal, neck extensors, and diaphragm

**What is the result of fatigable weakness of:**
    **Facial muscles?**

Flattened smile ("myasthenic snarl")

    **Bulbar muscles?**

Nasal speech, dysarthria, jaw fatigue, dysphagia

    **Neck extensors?**

Difficulty holding head up; patient may support head with hands

    **Diaphragm?**

Shortness of breath

**What is the distribution of limb weakness?**

Proximal > distal

**What is a myasthenic crisis?**

Severe respiratory muscle weakness requiring mechanical ventilation

**What is ocular myasthenia?**

Myasthenia gravis confined to extraocular and eyelid muscles

    **What percent of myasthenia gravis cases does it account for?**

15%

**What three tests are most useful in diagnosing myasthenia gravis?**

1. Tensilon (edrophonium) test
2. ACh receptor antibody
3. EMG/NCV

**What is the mechanism of action of Tensilon?**

It is an anticholinesterase that augments the neuromuscular transmitter ACh.

**How is a Tensilon test performed, and what happens?**

Ten mg of edrophonium is intravenously injected and briefly improves weakness in patients.

**What percentage of patients do not have ACh receptor antibodies?**

10–20% are "antibody negative"; the percentage is higher in ocular-only myasthenia.

**What special type of stimulation must be done during nerve conduction studies to diagnose myasthenia gravis?**

Repetitive nerve stimulation at slow rates (2–5 Hz)

**What does this show?**

Decrement of the response on successive stimulations, usually > 10% decrement in amplitude

**Why should chest CT be ordered when evaluating a patient with myasthenia gravis?**

The patient may have a hypertrophic thymus or thymoma.

**What surgical procedure is useful in the treatment of myasthenia gravis?**

Thymectomy–removal of normal, vestigial, or abnormal thymic tissue usually results in symptomatic improvement or even remission

**What are three types of therapy?**

1. Anticholinesterases [e.g., pyridostigmine (Mestinon)]
2. Immunosuppressants (e.g., prednisone, azathioprine)
3. Immunomodulation, with I.V.I.G., and plasma exchange

**Which therapy may initially exacerbate symptoms before improving them?**

Prednisone may exacerbate weakness during the first 1–2 weeks of treatment.

**What is a cholinergic crisis?**

Weakness due to anticholinergic drug overdose causing excessive ACh receptor-mediated depolarization

**Why is this a crisis?**

Oropharyngeal weakness increases the risk of aspiration.

| | |
|---|---|
| **What are four muscarinic symptoms of overdose in a cholinergic crisis?** | Salivation, abdominal cramps, nausea, vomiting |
| **What is the long-term prognosis of myasthenia gravis?** | Although respiratory distress may occur during acute exacerbations, the long-term prognosis is excellent, with negligible morbidity and mortality. |

## LAMBERT-EATON MYASTHENIC SYNDROME (LEMS)

| | |
|---|---|
| **Although rare, why is LEMS important to general physicians?** | 50% of cases are associated with malignancy |
| **With which malignancies is it associated?** | Lung, breast, prostate, stomach, rectum |
| **Which muscles are usually affected at presentation?** | Limb muscles |
| **How is this different from myasthenia gravis?** | Bulbar muscles are usually not involved in LEMS. |
| **Why is LEMS termed *myasthenic?*** | Weakness is fatigable. |
| **What systemic symptoms are usually present?** | Dry mouth, constipation, impotence and urinary difficulties due to autonomic dysfunction |
| **What is the fundamental defect in neuromuscular transmission?** | Presynaptic defect of ACh release due to antibody attack on N-M junction calcium channels |
| **Why does this cause systemic symptoms?** | The defect in neuromuscular transmission affects both nicotinic and muscarinic ACh receptors, resulting in autonomic dysfunction. |
| **What test distinguishes LEMS from myasthenia gravis?** | Repetitive nerve stimulation during EMG/NCV |
| **How?** | LEMS demonstrates *facilitation* (i.e., progressive increase in amplitude of the CMAP response) with repetitive |

stimulation at fast rates, whereas myasthenia gravis demonstrates *decremental response* (i.e., progressive decrease in amplitude) especially with slower rates of stimulation.

**What is the first step in management?**

Look for associated malignancy.

**What drugs may be useful in treatment of LEMS?**

Guanidine and diaminopyridine may improve weakness.

## OTHER DEFECTS OF NEUROMUSCULAR TRANSMISSION

**Name two acquired illnesses resulting from neuromuscular transmission defects.**

Botulism, curare poisoning

**How do they affect neuromuscular transmission?**

Botulinum toxin interferes with ACh release from presynaptic terminals. Curare blocks ACh receptors on muscle endplates.

# 15 _____

# Muscle Disorders
# (See Chapter 4)

| | |
|---|---|
| **What is a myopathy?** | Disease of muscle |
| **What is a myositis?** | Inflammatory disease of muscle |
| **What is muscular dystrophy?** | Progressive, genetically determined, non-inflammatory muscle cell loss |

## MYOPATHY

| | |
|---|---|
| **What is the location of weak muscles in myopathies?** | Proximal, greater than distal |
| **Describe the deep tendon reflexes in patients with myopathies.** | Present, but often decreased; commensurate with weakness |
| **What EMG findings suggest pathology in muscles?** | 1. Myopathic motor units, consisting of short duration, small amplitude motor units<br>2. Positive sharp waves<br>3. Fibrillation potentials in inflammatory myopathy (myositis) |
| **What is the single most important lab value in muscle diseases?** | Elevated creatine phosphokinase (CPK) |

## MYOSITIS (INFLAMMATORY MYOPATHY)

| | |
|---|---|
| **List three inflammatory myopathies.** | 1. Polymyositis<br>2. Dermatomyositis<br>3. Inclusion body myositis |
| **Is pain common in polymyositis?** | No. It occurs in about 15% of patients. |

**What percentage of patients with polymyositis have elevated ESR?**

About 50%

**What is the treatment of polymyositis?**

Corticosteroids, usually oral prednisone

**Is polymyositis associated with temporal (giant cell) arteritis?**

No, but polymyalgia rheumatica is

**Distinguish between polymyositis and dermatomyositis.**

Skin manifestations are present in dermatomyositis.

**What are the most frequent dermatologic findings in dermatomyositis?**

Purple or heliotrope rash of eyelids and periorbital edema

**Describe heliotrope.**

It is like a sunburn

**What systemic disease is associated with polymyositis and dermatomyositis in adults?**

Carcinoma—especially bronchogenic and colon in men and breast and ovarian in women

**What is the risk of occult carcinoma in adults with polymyositis or dermatomyositis?**

10–15%

**Describe dermatomyositis in children.**

Childhood dermatomyositis is more severe and painful than it is in adults, but associated neoplasia is very uncommon; childhood polymyositis is rare.

**What myopathy is suspect when a patient with myositis fails to improve on steroids?**

Inclusion body myositis

**How is it ruled out?**

Biopsy

## MYOTONIC DYSTROPHY

| | |
|---|---|
| **What is the appearance of patients with myotonic muscular dystrophy?** | Ptosis<br>Bifacial weakness<br>Frontal baldness (even in women)<br>Triangular face, giving a pouty or drooping, dull appearance |
| **What is the genetic defect and inheritance pattern in myotonic dystrophy?** | Trinucleotide repeat<br>Autosomal dominant<br>(See Table 48–1,K) |
| **What is the distribution of weakness?** | Distal greater than proximal, in contrast to other myopathic disorders |
| **What does myotonia look like on physical examination?** | Inability to relax a contracted muscle (e.g., patient is unable to let go after shaking hands) |
| **What is percussion myotonia?** | Contraction of a muscle in response to being tapped with percussion hammer; usually the thenar or hypothenar muscle of the hand or the tongue |
| **What does myotonia sound like on EMG?** | A dive-bomber sound that occurs as the muscle gradually relaxes after contraction or after movement of the recording needle |
| **What other organ is affected in almost all muscular dystrophies?** | The heart, especially in Duchenne and myotonic dystrophies |

## DUCHENNE MUSCULAR DYSTROPHY (See Chapter 4, Table 4–8)

| | |
|---|---|
| **What is the typical age of onset?** | Infancy or early childhood, around 3 to 6 years old |
| **What is the gender of the patients?** | Male |
| **Why?** | It is inherited as an X-linked recessive trait |
| **What is the biochemical defect?** | Absence of dystrophin, a structural muscle protein |

**What are the presenting symptoms?**

Proximal lower extremity (pelvic girdle and femoral) weakness with later involvement of upper extremity

**What is Gower's sign?**

It is the method by which patients overcome pelvic weakness when arising from a sitting position. They lean forward and brace the extended arms against the knees and "walk" their hands proximally up their thighs to straighten up.

**What is the distinctive characteristic of calf muscles?**

They are large due to "pseudohypertrophy" from infiltration by fibrous tissue and fat.

**What two tests are useful in diagnosis?**

CPK and EMG

**How is it definitively diagnosed?**

Muscle biopsy demonstrates absence of dystrophin protein.

**What is the time course of the weakness?**

Slowly progressive over many years

**What is the prognosis?**

Death usually occurs by 25 years of age because of respiratory or cardiac complications.

**Is any therapy useful?**

Oral steroids may slow progression of disease, but there is no curative therapy.

# 16

# Alcohol and the Nervous System

**What are six neurologic complications of alcoholism?**

Wernicke's encephalopathy, Korsakoff's syndrome, peripheral neuropathy (i.e., alcoholic polyneuropathy), seizures, cerebellar degeneration, dementia

**Why have Wernicke's encephalopathy and Korsakoff's syndrome traditionally been considered together?**

1. Both are alcohol-related confusional states.
2. Occasionally, they occur together in the same patient.

**Which is more common?**

Wernicke's encephalopathy

**What is it called when they occur together?**

Wernicke-Korsakoff syndrome

## WERNICKE'S ENCEPHALOPATHY

**What is the classic triad of signs in Wernicke's encephalopathy?**

Confusion, ataxia, and ophthalmoplegia

**What is the pathologic feature of Wernicke's encephalopathy?**

Periventricular degeneration, especially around the cerebral aqueduct and the third and fourth ventricles

**How is Wernicke's encephalopathy treated?**

Thiamine replacement

**Why is thiamine administered before glucose in a patient with altered consciousness?**

Administering glucose before thiamine may increase the risk of precipitously worsening the symptoms of Wernicke's encephalopathy.

## KORSAKOFF'S SYNDROME

| | |
|---|---|
| **What are the main features of Korsakoff's syndrome?** | Anterograde and retrograde amnesia; confabulation may be present |
| **What is the pathologic feature of Korsakoff's syndrome?** | Necrosis in selected areas of the thalamus and hypothalamus, most consistently in the mammillary bodies |
| **Is there any therapy available for Korsakoff's syndrome?** | No |

## ALCOHOLIC POLYNEUROPATHY

| | |
|---|---|
| **How does alcohol cause peripheral neuropathy?** | A toxic effect on nerves |
| **What are common presenting symptoms in an alcoholic polyneuropathy?** | Distal extremity pain, paresthesias, and weakness |
| **Characterize distal deep tendon reflexes in alcoholic polyneuropathy?** | As in all polyneuropathies, they are depressed or absent. |

## ALCOHOLIC CEREBELLAR DEGENERATION

| | |
|---|---|
| **What is the cardinal sign of alcoholic cerebellar degeneration?** | Ataxia of gait with relative sparing of upper extremity coordination |
| **What type of stance is observed in alcoholic cerebellar degeneration?** | Wide-based stance |
| **What is the cerebellar pathology?** | Degeneration of the superior anterior cerebellar vermis |

## ALCOHOL WITHDRAWAL SYNDROMES

| | |
|---|---|
| **What are the main symptoms of alcohol withdrawal?** | Nervousness, tremors, hallucinations, and seizures |

**When do alcohol withdrawal seizures occur in relation to the last drink?**

*Within* 2 days of the last drink

**When do the symptoms of delirium tremens appear in relation to the last drink?**

*After* 2 days from the last drink

**What are the six cardinal signs of delirium tremens?**

Confusion, agitation, insomnia, tremulousness, fever, and tachycardia

**How are alcohol withdrawal and delirium tremens treated?**

Benzodiazepines, usually diazepam (Valium), or chlordiazepoxide (Librium)

# Section III

Urgent Neurologic
Conditions

# 17

# Status Epilepticus

| | |
|---|---|
| **What is status epilepticus?** | A prolonged seizure or frequent repetitive seizures |
| **What are three categories of status epilepticus?** | 1. Generalized convulsive status epilepticus (GCSE)<br>2. Nonconvulsive status epilepticus<br>3. Simple partial status epilepticus, or epilepsia partialis continua (EPC) |

## GCSE

| | |
|---|---|
| **What is the formal definition of GCSE?** | A convulsion lasting greater than 30 minutes or recurrent convulsions over a 1-hour period without return of consciousness between seizures |
| **What is the incidence of GCSE?** | About 60,000 cases yearly in the United States |
| **What is the mortality from GCSE in the United States?** | About 10% |
| **What determines mortality in GCSE?** | The underlying etiology and the duration of the status epilepticus |
| **What is the most common etiology of GCSE?** | Patient noncompliance with anticonvulsant medication |
| **What are three other common etiologies of GCSE?** | Alcohol withdrawal, structural brain disease, systemic toxic and/or metabolic alterations |
| **Can GCSE be the initial presentation of epilepsy?** | Yes |
| **GCSE is most common in what age group?** | Children and elderly |

| | |
|---|---|
| **What are some systemic effects of GCSE on vital signs and blood chemistry?** | Temperature elevation, acidosis, hyperglycemia, hypertension |
| **What causes neuronal damage in GCSE?** | Prolonged and/or repeated depolarization of neurons |
| **What long-term sequelae may result from neuronal damage of GCSE?** | Future seizures, personality changes, and memory problems |

## TREATMENT

| | |
|---|---|
| **What principles guide treatment for GCSE?** | Protect the patient and stop the seizures. |
| **What should be done after termination?** | Search for and treat the etiology. |
| **What are some commonly used drugs in treatment of GCSE?** | Lorazepam, diazepam, fosphenytoin, phenytoin, and phenobarbital |
| **What is an appropriate loading dose of phenytoin or fosphenytoin?** | 15–20 mg/kg body weight |
| **What are two rate-limiting side effects of rapid use of phenytoin?** | Hypotension and bradycardia |
| **What is the fastest rate phenytoin can be given?** | 50 mg/min |
| **Why _shouldn't_ phenytoin be administered intramuscularly?** | Erratic rate of absorption |
| **What are three advantages of using fosphenytoin instead of phenytoin?** | 1. It may be administered at 150 mg/min with less hypotension or bradycardia<br>2. Less venous irritation<br>3. It can be administered intramuscularly |

**Other than administering anticonvulsants, what can be done to help terminate GCSE?**

Correct metabolic abnormalities if present

## NONCONVULSIVE STATUS EPILEPTICUS

**What is nonconvulsive status epilepticus?**

Recurring seizures without muscle contractions (i.e., convulsions)

**How does it usually present?**

Waxing and waning confusion or obtundation

**What is the diagnostic test for nonconvulsive status epilepticus?**

An electroencephalogram

**What are three other names that have been used for nonconvulsive status epilepticus?**

Ictal stupor, spike/wave stupor, absence status

## SIMPLE PARTIAL STATUS EPILEPTICUS

**What is another name for simple partial status epilepticus?**

Epilepsia partialis continua

**How does it usually present?**

Continuous jerking of a body part (e.g., a hand) with clear consciousness

**What is the most common EEG finding during EPC?**

Absence of EEG seizure activity despite clinical motor manifestations

**Is it more likely caused by a structural brain lesion or a systemic or metabolic disorder?**

Structural brain lesion

**How is it treated?**

With conventional anticonvulsants, but it is often refractory

# 18

# Brain Tumors

**Which is most common in adults, primary brain tumor or tumor that has metastasized to the brain?**

Tumor metastasized to the brain from some other location

**What are the three most common tumors that metastasize to the brain?**

Lung, melanoma, and breast: **L**ung **M**eets **B**rain

**Which is more likely to infiltrate surrounding brain tissue, primary or metastatic tumor?**

Primary

### Table 18–1. Brain Tumor Characteristics

| Tumor | Prognosis | Imaging Characteristics |
|---|---|---|
| Meningioma | No or slow growth | Dural, calcified, homogenous enhancement |
| Astrocytoma, grade I | Very slow growth | No edema; commonly enhance |
| Astrocytoma, grade II | 50% 5-year survival | Enhancement uncommon |
| Astrocytoma grade III | Median survival 2–3 years | May enhance |
| Glioblastoma multiforme | Rapidly growing, Median survival 10 months | Ring enhancement, edema |
| Oligodendroglioma | Variable, slow growing Median survival 10 years | Often calcified |
| Anaplastic oligodendroglioma | Median survival 4 years | Often enhance |
| Dysembryoplastic neuroepithelial tumor (DNET) | Very slow or no growth | Discrete increased homogeneous signal |
| Medulloblastoma | 60% curable with radio and chemotherapy | Cerebellum, primarily children |
| Primary CNS lymphoma | Median survival 3–4 years with chemoradiotherapy | Homogenous, sometimes multifocal enhancement |

## PRIMARY BRAIN TUMORS

| | |
|---|---|
| **Name the three most common primary parenchymal brain tumors.** | 1. Astrocytoma<br>2. Oligodendroglioma<br>3. Glioblastoma multiforme (considered very similar to a high-grade astrocytoma) |
| **State the relationship among their cells of origin.** | All arise from neuroglia. |
| **What is the most common malignant primary brain tumor?** | Glioblastoma multiforme |
| **Where are most primary brain tumors in adults located?** | Supratentorial region |
| **Is intracranial or intraspinal meningioma more common?** | Intracranial meningioma |
| **What tumor occurs in the retina and cerebellum as part of von Hippel-Lindau syndrome?** | Hemangioblastoma |
| **Is it familial?** | Yes |
| **Where are most primary brain tumors in children located?** | Infratentorial |
| **How common are CNS tumors among all childhood tumors?** | They are the most frequent solid neoplasm. |
| **What are the two most common brain tumors in children?** | Medulloblastoma and astrocytoma |

## SIGNS AND SYMPTOMS

| | |
|---|---|
| **How often do brain tumors present only with headache?** | Brain tumors rarely present only with headache. Headache is almost always accompanied by other features, such as mental status changes. |
| **Characterize the classic headache of a brain tumor.** | The headache is worst shortly after arising. |
| **Tinnitus, unilateral hearing loss, and vertigo are common presenting symptoms of which brain tumor?** | Acoustic schwannoma |
| **Which rare brain mass often causes symptoms of CSF obstruction when the person shifts head position?** | Colloid cyst of the third ventricle |

## DIAGNOSIS

| | |
|---|---|
| **What are two primary brain tumors that commonly show calcification on head CT?** | Meningioma and oligodendroglioma (low-grade astrocytoma occasionally is calcified) |
| **What is the typical appearance of glioblastoma multiforme on head CT?** | A heterogenous, or "messy" mass with surrounding edema, which may ring enhance with contrast |
| **Name four other lesions that may ring enhance.** | Brain abscess, metastatic tumor, toxoplasmosis, and lymphoma (in immunocompromised) |
| **What is the typical radiologic appearance of brain tumor of metastatic origin?** | Multiple lesions which enhance with contrast |
| **What are the two classic CSF abnormalities in brain tumor?** | Elevated pressure and protein |

**List four characteristics of brain tumor that may increase intracranial pressure.**

1. Space occupancy by the tumor itself
2. Edema of surrounding brain tissue
3. Obstruction of CSF pathways
4. Rarely, bleeding into the tumor

**How is a definitive diagnosis of a brain tumor made?**

Brain biopsy or resection, which usually identifies the cell type and differentiates tumor from abscess

## TREATMENT AND PROGNOSIS

**What options are available in the treatment of brain tumors?**

Steroids are useful in controlling cerebral edema.

Anticonvulsants can control seizures.

Surgical resection may be curative (or palliative by debulking).

Radiation therapy and gamma knife may cure some patients.

Chemotherapeutic agents are of benefit in many settings.

**What is the classic clinical course of brain tumor?**

Slow progression of focal neurologic deficit

# 19

# Brain Trauma

| | |
|---|---|
| **What is a closed head injury?** | Head trauma without skull fracture |
| **What are the most common brain injuries in closed head trauma?** | Contusion, subdural hematoma (SDH), traumatic subarachnoid hemorrhage (SAH), and diffuse axonal injury |
| **What is the term for a brief loss of consciousness after head trauma?** | Concussion |
| **What are the pathologic differences between a concussion and a contusion?** | Concussion: structural brain injury unlikely<br>Contusion: brain ecchymoses |
| **Where are cerebral contusions most often found?** | Frontal, occipital, and temporal poles |
| **What is "coup" and "contra-coup" brain injury?** | Contusion at site of head impact and contusion opposite to it, respectively |
| **What is the Munro-Kellie principle?** | The sum total of the mass of CSF, blood, and brain is a constant. To increase one of these three components will decrease another component or increase intracranial pressure (ICP). |
| **What scale is used in evaluation of head trauma?** | Glasgow Coma Scale |
| **What are the three components of the Glasgow Coma Scale?** | 1. Verbal responsiveness<br>2. Motor responsiveness<br>3. Eye opening response |
| **How does the Glasgow Coma Scale aid patient management?** | It permits a quick, objective rating of brain function from one evaluation to the next. |

| How is it scored? | Scores range from 3 (no responses) to 15 (normal) |
|---|---|

**Table 19–1.    Glasgow Coma Scale Scoring**

| Category | Points for a Given Response |
|---|---|
| Motor response | 6—Obeys verbal command to move<br>5—Localizes (i.e., moves hand to) painful stimuli<br>4—Withdraws arm from stimulus<br>3—Stimulus causes flexion posturing<br>2—Stimulus causes extension posturing<br>1—No response |
| Verbal response | 5—Fully oriented<br>4—Not fully oriented<br>3—Verbalizes, but not normally conversant<br>2—Vocalizes unintelligible sounds<br>1—No vocalization |
| Eye opening | 4—Spontaneously opens eyes<br>3—Opens eyes to speech<br>2—Opens eyes to painful stimulus<br>1—No eye opening |

| **What are four signs of basilar skull fracture?** | Hemotympanum, raccoon's eyes (periorbital ecchymoses), Battle's sign (postauricular ecchymoses), CSF rhinorrhea/otorrhea |
|---|---|
| **Which cranial nerves are most commonly affected by basilar skull fracture?** | Facial (CN VII)<br>Vestibulocochlear (CN VIII) |
| **What is the first sign of increased ICP secondary to trauma?** | Decreased level of consciousness |
| **What are the three classic signs of Cushing's triad of ICP?** | Hypertension, bradycardia, respiratory irregularity |
| **Why does transtentorial herniation cause a dilated pupil?** | Pressure on CN III or brain stem from which it originates |
| **What is the differential diagnosis for a single dilated pupil in evaluation of a closed head injury?** | Transtentorial herniation<br>Carotid-cavernous sinus fistula<br>Traumatic CN III injury |

| | |
|---|---|
| **What complication of closed head injury should be suspected in a patient with proptosis, retro-orbital pain, and ocular bruit?** | Carotid-cavernous sinus fistula |

## MANAGEMENT OF A CLOSED HEAD INJURY

| | |
|---|---|
| **How early should you feed someone after severe closed head injury?** | As soon as possible, TPN if necessary |
| **Are steroids useful in the management of severe closed head injury?** | No |
| **What are the most common late complications of head injury?** | Postconcussive syndrome, seizure, cognitive impairment |
| **List four components of the postconcussive syndrome.** | Headache, dizziness, psychologic disorders, cognitive impairment |
| **What are the cardinal features of "dementia pugilistica," associated with boxing?** | Dysarthria, parkinsonism, dementia |
| **What causes a knockout in boxing?** | Probably brain stem concussion, perhaps followed by brain stem contusion or laceration when the head strikes the mat |

## EPIDURAL HEMATOMA

| | |
|---|---|
| **In closed head injury, what is the significance of progressive coma and lateralizing signs after a lucid interval?** | May indicate an expanding mass, such as an epidural hematoma |
| **Trauma to what vessel most commonly causes epidural hematoma?** | Middle meningeal artery |

| | |
|---|---|
| **What additional injury should always be suspected in a patient with a temporal skull fracture?** | Epidural hematoma caused by laceration of underlying middle meningeal artery |
| **What is the classic CT finding of epidural hematoma?** | Convex hyperdensity outside brain tissue in parietotemporal region |
| **What is the mortality in untreated epidural hematoma?** | Almost 100% |

## SDH

| | |
|---|---|
| **Trauma to what vessels is most often related to SDH?** | "Bridging veins" between inner and outer meningeal membranes. |
| **In what age group are chronic SDHs usually seen?** | The elderly |
| **Why does an SDH usually accumulate more slowly than an epidural hematoma?** | Because the subdural is of venous origin, whereas the epidural is arterial |
| **What is the classic CT finding of SDH?** | Crescent-shaped hyperintensity between brain and skull |
| **What is an excessive collection of CSF in the subdural space termed?** | Subdural hygroma |

## DEFINITIONS

**Define coma.**

Unresponsiveness to external or internal stimuli

**Define altered mental state.**

Any decreased consciousness or confusion

**Define consciousness.**

Appropriate awareness of the environment

**Is it wise to use the terms *stupor* and *lethargy*?**

These terms are imprecise; it is better to describe the patient.

## THE ANATOMIC BASIS OF COMA

**Localize the lesion in the nervous system producing coma.**

Either **both** cerebral hemispheres or the reticular activating system (RAS) [i.e., upper brain stem or diencephalon]

**Can stroke cause coma?**

In the brain stem, yes. In the cerebral hemisphere, no (unless there is brain swelling with compression of the opposite hemisphere or brain stem).

**Can unilateral cerebral hemisphere disease cause coma?**

No–it must be both hemispheres

**What is the RAS?**

A diffuse collection of neurons in the upper brain stem (i.e., upper pons, midbrain, and diencephalon)

**What does the RAS do?**

It is the main structure responsible for alertness and arousal.

## EVALUATION OF THE COMATOSE PATIENT

**What is the Glasgow Coma Scale?**

A scoring system based on a brief neurologic examination used to assess mental status and predict outcome in coma following head trauma (see Chapter 18)

**What are four important bedside clinical tests for brain stem function in a comatose patient?**

1. Pupillary light reflex
2. Corneal response
3. Oculocephalic response (doll's eyes)
4. Caloric response (vestibulo-ocular reflex)

**What is a "blown pupil?"**

A dilated pupil unreactive to light stimulation

**What does it indicate?**

Usually pressure on brain stem or ipsilateral third cranial nerve from brain displaced by increased ICP

**What are doll's eyes?**

The oculocephalic, or cervico-ocular, reflex. In coma with an intact brain stem, rotating the patient's head one way causes the eyes to deviate in the opposite direction, followed immediately by return to midposition. This is sometimes called a positive doll's eyes.

**Explain the neuroanatomic basis of doll's eyes.**

Rotation initiates signals from neck stretch receptors that are conducted to CN III, IV, and VI through a healthy brain stem (see Chapter 3).

**What is the significance of absent doll's eyes in coma?**

It indicates either a damaged brain stem or diffuse cerebral dysfunction.

**Do awake, normal people have doll's eyes present?**

No. Awake people with an intact cortex have the ability to overcome the deviation of the eyes.

**What are cold calorics?**

The vestibulo-ocular reflex. With an intact brain stem, cold water lavage of the ear causes the eyes to *deviate (gaze) toward* the cold water. In an awake person, this test induces nystagmus with the fast component in the opposite direction of gaze deviation.

**What response indicates a brain stem lesion?**

Lack of or incomplete gaze deviation

**What does the mnemonic COWS stand for?**

Cold-**O**pposite, **W**arm-**S**ame: This refers to the fast phase of the nystagmus when the cerebral cortex is in control of the brain stem. Note that this does not refer to the direction of gaze deviation.

**What does the presence of COWS indicate?**

Presence of nystagmus is proof that the patient is not comatose.

**What are decerebrate and decorticate responses?**

Responses of a comatose patient to noxious stimulation

**Distinguish between them.**

In decorticate (or flexor) posturing, the arms flex, bringing the hands close to the heart, or "*cor*."

In decerebrate (or extensor) posturing, the arms extend.

**What is the physiologic basis of decorticate and decerebrate posturing?**

Decorticate posturing indicates dysfunction above the red nucleus in the midbrain, so rubrospinal function continues. Decerebrate posturing indicates a lesion of brain stem between red and vestibular nuclei with loss of rubrospinal function; the patient displays the increased tone of unopposed vestibulospinal system.

**Restate their anatomic localization in relation to whole brain versus cerebral cortex.**

Decorticate posturing indicates a lesion immediately below the *cortex*, in the white matter of the cerebral hemispheres or the uppermost brain stem.

Decerebrate posturing indicates a lower lesion. It is below the whole *cerebrum*, in the midbrain or pons.

**Which lesion is higher in the brain stem, and how can you remember this?**

The cortex is "higher" than the cerebrum; therefore, decortication indicates a higher lesion than decerebration.

**Localize the level of the lesion causing these respiratory patterns:**
  **Post-hyperventilation apnea?**

Bilateral hemispheres

| | |
|---|---|
| **Cheyne-Stokes respiration?** | Bilateral hemispheres |
| **Central reflex hyperpnea?** | Lower midbrain–upper pons (central neurogenic hyperventilation) |
| **Apneustic breathing?** | Mid-pons |
| **Cluster breathing (Biot)?** | Medulla |
| **Apnea?** | Medulla |

## MANAGEMENT AND PROGNOSIS OF THE COMATOSE PATIENT

| | |
|---|---|
| **What are the first steps in the management of a newly comatose patient?** | As with all unconscious patients:<br>**A**irway<br>**B**reathing<br>**C**irculation<br>Then search out and treat the underlying cause |
| **What lab tests should be ordered and why?** | Blood chemistry: abnormal glucose or sodium levels<br>Toxicology screen: alcohol, drugs of abuse, other toxins<br>ABG: hypoxia, hypercarbia<br>CBC: low hematocrit with hemorrhagic shock; high or low WBC in sepsis<br>Blood cultures: if sepsis is suspected<br>Head CT: intracranial hemorrhage; large ischemic stroke<br>Lumbar puncture: if CNS infection is suspected |
| **What CSF pressure level constitutes increased ICP?** | 18 cm of water or more on lumbar puncture in lateral recumbent position |
| **What medications should be administered to a newly comatose patient?** | Naloxone (Narcan), which is an opiate antagonist<br>D-50 (dextrose and water), which is used to treat possible hypoglycemia<br>Thiamine, which is used to prevent Wernicke's encephalopathy |

| | |
|---|---|
| **What four features of the neurologic examination best aid management and prognosis?** | Alertness, pupillary responses, eye movements, and posturing |

## THE LOCKED-IN PATIENT

| | |
|---|---|
| **What is the locked-in state?** | An alert patient who is unable to move, except eyes and upper eyelids |
| **Why is a locked-in patient mistakenly thought to be comatose?** | Although alert to a normal degree, all muscles except for the eyes are paralyzed. |
| **What is its etiology?** | Usually, infarction of all voluntary motor pathways in base of pons except those that have already innervated CN III in the midbrain. Consciousness is not involved. |

## PERSISTENT VEGETATIVE STATE

| | |
|---|---|
| **What is persistent vegetative state?** | The person is awake but unaware of self or environment. |
| **How long must it persist to justify the diagnosis?** | 1 month |
| **Localize the lesion in persistent vegetative state.** | Cerebral cortex, sparing brain stem |
| **What are four intact functions in this state?** | Sleep–wake cycles, eye opening, eye tracking, swallowing |
| **What functions are absent?** | Speech and responses to command or noxious stimuli |
| **How long must it persist before it becomes permanent?** | After trauma—at least 12 months<br>After anoxia—at least 3 months; some studies suggest even longer before it is irreversible |

## ELEVATED INTRACRANIAL PRESSURE (ICP)

| | |
|---|---|
| **Excess of any of what three intracranial substances results in elevated ICP?** | 1. Brain parenchyma (e.g., edema)<br>2. CSF (e.g., hydrocephalus)<br>3. Blood (e.g., SDH) |

| | |
|---|---|
| **State two ways in which elevated ICP injures brain function.** | 1. It decreases cerebral blood flow.<br>2. It injures the brain stem by brain displacement. |
| **What is the first sign of acutely elevated ICP?** | Decreased level of consciousness |
| **What are two signs of herniation of the temporal lobe (uncus) through the tentorial notch (transtentorial herniation)?** | 1. Dilated pupil caused by dysfunction of CN III<br>2. Hemiparesis caused by pressure on the cerebral peduncle |
| **What are three important signs of cerebellar tonsil herniation?** | 1. Respiratory arrest<br>2. Bradycardia<br>3. Hypertension |
| **What causes them?** | Lower medullary compression |

ICP MONITORING

| | |
|---|---|
| **What is normal ICP?** | Less than 15 torr (mm Hg) |
| **When is ICP monitoring indicated?** | Trauma with decreased level of consciousness<br>Reye's syndrome<br>Any time elevated ICP suspected |
| **What are two methods of ICP monitoring?** | Intraventricular catheter<br>Intraparenchymal fiberoptic pressure monitor (Camino catheter)<br>(Subdural and epidural monitoring systems are also available.) |

TREATMENT

| | |
|---|---|
| **What are four non-drug therapies for elevated ICP?** | 1. Elevate head above heart<br>2. Keep head in midline to avoid pressure on jugular veins, which can elevate intracranial venous pressure<br>3. Hyperventilate to keep $Pco_2$ 25–30 mm Hg<br>4. Remove CSF by ventriculostomy |
| **What are three drug therapies for elevated ICP?** | 1. 25% mannitol (about 0.5 mg/kg, or 50–100 g in an adult) to osmotically draw fluid from brain<br>2. Steroids to decrease vasogenic edema |

3. High-dose barbiturates to reduce cerebral blood volume

**What surgical option, other than ventriculostomy and drainage of CSF, is available for treatment of elevated ICP?**

Hemicraniectomy (i.e., removal of part of the skull)

# 21

# Brain Death

## DEFINITIONS

| | |
|---|---|
| **What is the clinical definition of brain death?** | Absence of response to external stimuli due to permanent destruction of both cerebral hemispheres and brain stem |
| **Distinguish brain death from coma.** | Brain death is irreversible. Coma is unconsciousness that may be reversible. |
| **What is consciousness?** | Appropriate awareness of the environment |

## CRITERIA

| | |
|---|---|
| **How long must coma last before brain death is considered?** | Usually 6 hours, but depending on state law, may be up to 24 hours |
| **What historical point must be documented to declare a brain as dead?** | The absence of sedative drug administration |
| **What vital signs must be normal to declare brain death?** | **Temperature**—severe hypothermia can mimic brain death and is potentially reversible<br>**Blood pressure**—adult systolic pressure > 80 mm Hg |
| **What evaluation must precede consideration of brain death?** | Reversible causes of coma, including structural lesions, metabolic, and infectious causes (see Chapter 19), must be excluded. |
| **What empiric drug trials may help exclude reversible causes of coma?** | Administration of:<br>1. Thiamine and glucose for alcoholic hypoglycemia<br>2. Naloxone for narcotics<br>3. Flumazenil for benzodiazepine overdosage |

## PHYSICAL EXAMINATION OF BRAIN DEATH

**How is brain death demonstrated on neurologic exam?**

It is demonstrated by the absence of cortical and brain stem responses.

**What are four cranial nerve reflexes that are tested in brain death?**

1. Pupillary responses
2. Corneal reflexes
3. Gag reflex
4. Vestibulo-ocular reflex (cold calorics)

**What are the pupillary findings in brain death?**

"Fixed" pupils unresponsive to light that are dilated or in midposition

**What four common classes of medications can cause fixed or nearly fixed pupils?**

1. Ophthalmoplegics (e.g., atropine)
2. Systemic anticholinergics
3. Neuromuscular blockers
4. Sedatives

**What is the quick-and-dirty eye test of brain stem function?**

The doll's eye test

**How is it done?**

Rapidly rotate head of unconscious patient; observe eyes

**What response indicates normal brain stem function?**

Conjugate deviation of both eyes opposite to head rotation.

**What examination technique is used to test vestibulo-ocular reflexes?**

Cold water calorics

**What three common classes of medications can obliterate responses to cold calorics by causing ophthalmoplegia?**

Neuromuscular blockers, sedatives, and anticonvulsants (e.g., phenobarbital, phenytoin, carbamazepine) in toxic doses

**How do you test motor responses in an unconscious patient?**

Withdrawal to painful stimuli, such as pinch or pressure

**What activity may persist despite brain death?**

Deep tendon reflexes or pathologic spinal reflexes, such as triple flexion

**What test excludes spontaneous breathing?**

Apnea test

**How is the apnea test performed?**

The patient is ventilated for 10 minutes with 100% oxygen to raise $PaO_2$ to supramaximal levels. Ventilation is then stopped, and oxygen via tracheal tube is suffused at 6 lpm to maintain normal $PaO_2$. $PaCO_2$ should rise 3 mm Hg/min. If after 10 minutes the patient has not breathed and the $PaCO_2 \geq 60$ mm Hg, then the respiratory center at the level of the medulla is not functional.

**When is physical examination insufficient to diagnose brain death?**

When confounding factors exist, including presence of sedative medications, hypothermia, or when the patient is not medically stable enough for the apnea test

## CONFIRMATORY TESTS

**What three confirmatory tests are useful in evaluation of brain death?**

EEG, radionuclide cerebral perfusion scan, and cerebral angiography

**What findings on EEG support brain death?**

Isoelectric EEG, recorded during 30 minutes, with specific techniques for evaluating brain death

**What findings on cerebral perfusion scan and cerebral arteriography confirm the diagnosis?**

Lack of cerebral blood flow

**What are the pathologic findings of brain death on autopsy?**

Widespread CNS softening and necrosis ("respirator brain")

**What are you required to ask family members once brain death has been established?**

Organ procurement. Most states have wallet cards attached to drivers' licenses. These cards supersede family members' permission.

**Make a table of clinical examination and confirmatory test results in brain death.**

### Table 21–1. Diagnosis of Brain Death

| Diagnostic Tests | Result |
|---|---|
| **Clinical Examination** | |
| Illuminate pupils | No pupilloconstriction |
| Touch corneas | No blink |
| Doll's eyes | No response |
| Cold calorics | No response |
| Painful stimulation | No response |
| Apnea test | No respiratory effort |
| **Confirmatory Tests** | |
| EEG | Isoelectric (Flat line) |
| Carotid arteriography or radionuclide scan | No cerebral blood flow |
| Pharmacologic tests | |
| Glucose and thiamine | For hypoglycemia |
| Narcan | For narcotics |
| Flumazenil | For benzodiazepines |

# 22

# Infections

## MENINGITIS

| | |
|---|---|
| **What are the three major groups of pathogens that cause meningitis?** | Bacteria, viruses, and fungi |
| **What are the five most common bacterial pathogens that cause meningitis?** | 1. *Streptococcus pneumoniae*<br>2. *Neisseria meningitidis*<br>3. *Haemophilus influenzae*<br>4. *Escherichia coli*<br>5. *Listeria monocytogenes* |

**What pathogens are classically associated with bacterial meningitis:**

| | |
|---|---|
| **In neonates?** | Group B streptococcus, *E. coli* |
| **In children?** | *S. pneumoniae* is the most important cause, because now most children in the United States are immunized against *H. influenzae,* which was previously common. |
| **In adults?** | *S. pneumoniae, N. meningitidis* |
| **In the elderly?** | *L. monocytogenes, S. pneumoniae* |
| **What are the most common symptoms of meningitis?** | Stiff neck (nuchal rigidity), headache, fever, vomiting, confusion, seizures |
| **Name two signs associated with meningeal irritation.** | Kernig's and Brudzinski's signs |
| **What is Kernig's sign?** | With patient supine, examiner flexes patient's hip, but cannot extend the knee without causing neck pain and flexion. (Remember: **K**ernig's=**K**nee.) |

**What is Brudzinski's sign?**

Flexion of the neck causes flexion of the legs at the knees, hips, and ankles.

**What is the test of choice for diagnosing meningitis?**

Evaluation of CSF

**What are the risks of lumbar puncture (LP) or spinal tap?**

Small risk of infection, bleeding, or brain herniation

**How can one reduce the risk of herniation from an LP?**

Before performing LP, check for papilledema or other focal neurologic signs that suggest elevated ICP.

**If there is papilledema or other focal neurologic signs, what other test should be performed before LP?**

Head CT to look for hydrocephalus, mass-occupying lesion, or cerebral edema

**Is herniation likely in meningitis? Why?**

It is unlikely because the process is diffuse and located superficially in the meninges.

**What are the most common CSF findings in bacterial meningitis?**

Highly increased WBC (**neutrophils** predominate), increased protein, decreased glucose, increased opening pressure; CSF cultures positive in 75% of cases

**What are the most common CSF findings in viral meningitis?**

Slightly increased WBC (**lymphocytes** predominate), mildly elevated protein, normal glucose

**What are the most common CSF findings in fungal meningitis?**

Moderately increased WBC (**lymphocytes** predominate), increased protein, decreased glucose

**What are the most common CSF findings in tuberculous meningitis?**

Variably increased WBC (lymphocytes), moderately decreased glucose, very high protein

**Chart the CSF findings in bacterial, viral, fungal, and tuberculous meningitis.**

**Table 22–1.   CSF Findings in Acute Meningitis**

| Type | Pleocytosis | Glucose | Protein |
|------|-------------|---------|---------|
| Bacterial | ↑↑↑ (Neutrophils) | ↓↓↓ | ↑↑ |
| Viral | ↑ (Lymphocytes) | nl | ↑ |
| Fungal | ↑↑ (Lymphocytes) | ↓ | ↑ |
| Tuberculous | ↑ (Lymphocytes) | ↓↓ | ↑↑↑ |

↑ = increased; ↓ = decreased. (See also Chapter 44, Lumbar Puncture and CSF Analysis.)

**What conditions predispose patients to meningitis?**

Infection: systemic (particularly respiratory) and parameningeal
Head trauma
Neurosurgical procedures
Cancer
Alcoholism
Immunodeficiency
Absence of spleen

**What is the empiric treatment for bacterial meningitis?**

Antibiotics based on patient's age and suspected organism

**What empiric antibiotics are most appropriate in an adult with meningitis?**

Third-generation cephalosporins (e.g., ceftriaxone) and ampicillin. If cephalosporin/penicillin–resistant pneumococcus is prominent, then vancomycin should be added. A third-generation cephalosporin should still be used because vancomycin has poor CNS penetration.

**Is there a role for corticosteroids in the treatment of meningitis?**

Yes, but it is controversial. It can reduce the risk of hearing loss in children.

**When should corticosteroids be given?**

Before or with antibiotics, but antibiotics should never be delayed because of corticosteroid use

| | |
|---|---|
| **What is the mortality of bacterial meningitis?** | Varies with etiologic agent:<br>   25% die with pneumococcus<br>   10% die with meningococcus<br>   5% die with *H. influenzae* |
| **What is aseptic meningitis?** | Meningitis in which the pathogen cannot be identified; usually there is CSF lymphocytic pleocytosis and normal glucose |
| **What is the most common presumptive cause of aseptic meningitis?** | Usually a virus |

## FUNGAL MENINGITIS

| | |
|---|---|
| **What is the most common etiology of fungal meningitis?** | Cryptococcus |
| **What other form of meningitis does the clinical presentation resemble?** | Aseptic meningitis |
| **What is the most common risk factor for fungal meningitis?** | Immunodeficiency, especially HIV infection |
| **What laboratory tests rapidly identify cryptococci in CSF?** | India ink stain of CSF and cryptococcal antigen tests |
| **What is the conventional treatment?** | Amphotericin B. In HIV patients, prolonged therapy with an oral antifungal (e.g., fluconazole) is often required to suppress chronic infection. |

## TUBERCULOUS (TB) MENINGITIS

| | |
|---|---|
| **What are some common risk factors for TB meningitis?** | History of pulmonary TB, alcoholism, corticosteroid use, HIV, impaired immune response, resident of endemic area or group |
| **What organism usually causes tuberculous meningitis?** | *Mycobacterium tuberculosis*; rarely, *Mycobacterium bovis* |

**Is TB meningitis usually a primary infection or reactivation of a previous infection?**

Usually reactivation of previous infection

**In what percentage of patients with TB meningitis is there active pulmonary TB?**

Approximately 66%

**What are the symptoms and signs of TB meningitis?**

Fever, confusion, headache, nuchal rigidity (75% of cases)

**Over what period of time do the symptoms of TB meningitis develop?**

Approximately 2 weeks (compared with hours to days for typical bacterial meningitis)

**What is the most remarkable CSF finding in TB meningitis?**

Markedly increased CSF protein; acid-fast bacilli are rarely seen

**How long does it take to culture *M. tuberculosis*?**

Up to 1 month—as much CSF as possible must be submitted to the lab because there are usually very few tubercle bacilli.

**What are the pathologic findings seen in TB meningitis?**

Exudate in subarachnoid space, especially at base of brain with inflammation of:
Adjacent brain (basal meningoencephalitis)
Cranial nerves (causing cranial neuropathies)
Arteries (arteritis and possible thrombosis)
Basal cisterns (obstruction and possible hydrocephalus)

**What are the imaging findings in TB meningitis?**

Enhancement of basal cisterns and meninges; hydrocephalus

**What is the prognosis of TB meningitis?**

10–33% of patients die despite appropriate treatment

**What is the most significant predictor of a poor outcome?**

Coma at time of presentation

| | |
|---|---|
| **What is the natural history of untreated TB meningitis?** | Confusion progressing to stupor and coma, with cranial nerve palsies, elevated intracerebral pressure, decerebrate posturing, and death in 1–2 months |
| **Which age groups are at greatest risk?** | Youngest and oldest |

## HERPES SIMPLEX VIRUS (HSV) ENCEPHALITIS

| | |
|---|---|
| **What age groups are most susceptible to HSV encephalitis?** | All ages<br>Adults, especially HSV-1<br>Neonates, especially HSV-2 |
| **Are there seasons or geographic areas of increased risk?** | No |
| **What is the approximate annual incidence of HSV encephalitis in the United States?** | Approximately 2,000 cases per year |
| **List the three most frequent presenting complaints.** | 1. Headache<br>2. Change in mental status<br>3. Seizures |
| **Do adults with HSV encephalitis usually have oral or genital herpes?** | Neither |
| **What three tests are helpful in the diagnosis of HSV encephalitis?** | LP, EEG, MRI |
| **What are the most common findings on these tests?** | LP: elevated opening pressure; pleocytosis (lymphocytes) often with RBCs; increased protein; normal glucose (similar to viral meningitis)<br>EEG: periodic lateralizing epileptiform discharges (PLEDS)<br>MRI: Focal area T2 high signal, usually of the temporal lobes, with gadolinium enhancement |

| How can the diagnosis of HSV be definitively ascertained? | Brain biopsy or PCR test for herpes organisms in CSF |
|---|---|
| What are the pathologic changes? | Gross: hemorrhagic necrosis of frontal and temporal lobes<br>Microscopic: necrosis and inflammation with eosinophilic intranuclear inclusion bodies |
| What is the treatment for HSV encephalitis? | Intravenous acyclovir |
| What is an avoidable complication of acyclovir? | Renal impairment, usually avoided by hydration and usually reversible |
| What is the morbidity and mortality of HSV encephalitis? | Untreated cases: 33–75% die within 18 months<br>Treated cases: survival increases up to 90% with the use of acyclovir |
| What are the most common sequelae? | Memory and behavior problems |

## HIV

| What are the three central nervous system diseases caused specifically by HIV? | 1. HIV meningitis<br>2. Vacuolar myelopathy<br>3. AIDS dementia complex (ADC) |
|---|---|
| What are the three peripheral nervous system locations directly affected by HIV? | 1. Muscles (myopathy)<br>2. Nerves (neuropathy)<br>3. Nerve roots (radiculopathy) |
| List some common secondary viral, bacterial, and fungal agents that infect the CNS in AIDS patients. | Cytomegalovirus, HSV, varicella-zoster virus, JC virus (progressive multifocal leukoencephalopathy), tuberculosis, neurosyphilis, toxoplasma, cryptococcus |
| What is the most common CNS complication of HIV? | ADC |

## HIV MENINGITIS

| | |
|---|---|
| **What are the clinical characteristics of primary HIV meningitis?** | Indistinguishable from any other aseptic meningitis |
| **When does HIV meningitis usually occur in the course of HIV disease?** | Around the time of seroconversion |
| **What are the CSF characteristics of HIV meningitis?** | Mild CSF lymphocytosis and protein elevation, similar to aseptic meningitis |
| **How is it treated?** | Highly active antiretroviral therapy (HAART) consisting of combinations of agents |

## AIDS DEMENTIA COMPLEX (ADC)

| | |
|---|---|
| **What are the early symptoms and signs in ADC?** | Cortical dysfunction: memory loss, behavioral change, impaired motor skills<br>Subcortical white matter dysfunction: UMN signs<br>Cerebellar dysfunction: ataxia, postural tremor |
| **What are the common late symptoms and signs in ADC?** | Dementia, psychosis, seizures, incontinence, spastic paralysis |
| **What are the typical CSF findings in ADC?** | Mild CSF lymphocytosis, increased protein, sometimes oligoclonal bands |
| **What do imaging studies in ADC demonstrate?** | Cerebral atrophy, ventricular dilation, subcortical white matter disease (suggesting demyelination) |
| **What is the treatment for ADC?** | HAART |
| **What is the prognosis and clinical course in ADC?** | Progressive decline to death within 1 year, usually because of secondary infections; however, HAART therapy reduces progression to ADC by approximately 50% |

| | |
|---|---|
| **What are some of the neurologic adverse effects of AZT?** | Headache, generalized weakness and fatigue, myalgia and mitochondrial myopathy |

## HIV VACUOLAR MYELOPATHY

| | |
|---|---|
| **What is HIV vacuolar myelopathy?** | Vacuolar degeneration of spinal cord white matter |
| **What is its prevalence?** | It is found at autopsy in about 25% of AIDS patients. |
| **What are the most common signs and symptoms of vacuolar myelopathy?** | Like other myelopathies; motor and sensory deficits as well as incontinence |
| **What other HIV neurologic disease is comorbid with vacuolar myelopathy?** | ADC |
| **What are the MRI findings in vacuolar myelopathy?** | Typically normal |
| **What is the major differential diagnosis of vacuolar myelopathy?** | Vitamin $B_{12}$ myelopathy, which also affects corticospinal and posterior columns |
| **Is its course different?** | Vacuolar myelopathy usually has an earlier onset of incontinence and fewer sensory abnormalities. |

## MUSCLE AND PERIPHERAL NERVE DISEASES IN AIDS

| | |
|---|---|
| **How common is peripheral nerve disease in AIDS patients?** | About 50% of AIDS patients have pathology of peripheral nerves at autopsy. |
| **Specify the four most common peripheral nerve diseases in patients with AIDS?** | Sensorimotor polyneuropathy<br>Chronic inflammatory demyelinating polyneuropathy (CIDP)<br>Lumbosacral polyradiculopathy<br>Mononeuritis multiplex |
| **What is the most common myopathy associated with AIDS?** | HIV polymyositis |

| | |
|---|---|
| **What is the clinical presentation of HIV polymyositis?** | Similar to other polymyositis (i.e., trunk and proximal limb weakness) |
| **What is the treatment for HIV polymyositis?** | Corticosteroids |

## TOXOPLASMOSIS IN AIDS

| | |
|---|---|
| **What is the differential diagnosis for a solitary brain lesion on MRI in an AIDS patient?** | Toxoplasmosis, primary CNS lymphoma, brain abscess |
| **How can you differentiate CNS toxoplasmosis from primary CNS lymphoma?** | Radiologically they may be identical. Treat for toxoplasmosis. If no regression in the size of lesion, brain biopsy is necessary. |

## PROGRESSIVE MULTIFOCAL LEUKOENCEPHALOPATHY (PML)

| | |
|---|---|
| **What is the causative agent of PML?** | JC virus—a polyoma virus that is a subgroup of papovaviruses |
| **Where did the virus' name come from?** | The afflicted patient's initials |
| **What concurrent medical condition predisposes a patient to the development of PML?** | Immunocompromise (e.g., HIV, chronic steroid use, leukemia) |
| **What cells does it affect?** | Oligodendroglia and astroglia |
| **Based on what you should know about which cells are affected in PML, what would you expect to see on MRI?** | Multiple focal lesions in white matter (this is the origin of its name) |
| **What are three common clinical findings in patients with PML?** | Mental or personality changes, paresis, ataxia |
| **What are the treatments available for PML?** | None are effective, although ganciclovir and others have been tried. |

# CREUTZFELDT-JAKOB DISEASE (CJD)

| | |
|---|---|
| **Who gets CJD?** | Adults |
| **Is it caused by the JC virus?** | No |
| **What is the causative agent?** | It is a prion disease. |
| **What is its mechanism of disease?** | It converts amyloid to beta-pleated sheets, which deposit in the brain. |
| **What is a prion?** | Small, infectious, proteinaceous particle |
| **How is this agent transmitted?** | Usually by exposure to infected material, but may occur sporadically |
| **In the past, what patients have been particularly at risk?** | Recipients of corneal and organ transplants as well as human pituitary growth hormone |
| **What is its neuropathologic picture?** | Spongiform encephalopathy |
| **What does a spongiform encephalopathy look like microscopically?** | Gliosis, loss of neurons and vacuolization of background |
| **What is the predominant presenting symptom of patients with CJD?** | Rapidly progressing dementia |
| **What is the classic triad of findings in CJD?** | Dementia, myoclonus, characteristic EEG findings |
| **What is the classic EEG finding?** | Periodic generalized high-amplitude sharp wave complexes that may correlate with myoclonic jerks |
| **What are three features that frequently occur at some point in its course?** | Myoclonic jerks, visual hallucinations, ataxia |
| **What is the treatment of CJD?** | There is none. |

**What is its prognosis?**

Invariably fatal

**What is the limitation caused by CJD on organ donor recruitment?**

Donors may not be demented or have received transplants.

**What is the name of a similar disease that was found among natives of New Guinea?**

Kuru

**What was its method of person to person transmission?**

Ritual cannibalism

**What is the name of a similar infectious spongioform neurodegenerative disease found in sheep?**

Scrapie

**What is the name of a similar infectious spongioform neurodegenerative disease of cattle**

BSE (bovine spongioform encephalopathy)

**Is it transmissable to humans?**

Yes

**What is its vernacular name?**

Mad cow disease

**What is the three-German eponym of another human subacute spongioform encephalopathy often due to inherited genetic abnormality?**

Gerstmann-Straussler-Scheinker disease

# Section IV

## Other Important Neurologic Conditions

# 23    Amyotrophic Lateral Sclerosis

| | |
|---|---|
| **What is the eponym for amyotrophic lateral sclerosis (ALS)?** | Lou Gehrig's disease |
| **What are the different varieties of ALS?** | Most cases are sporadic, but there are familial forms and also overlap syndromes of ALS plus parkinsonism and dementia. The latter predominantly occur in Guam, New Guinea, and Japan. |
| **What is the most common variety of ALS?** | Sporadic; only about 10% of cases are familial |
| **What inheritance pattern does familial ALS follow?** | Autosomal dominant |
| **For what product does the gene encode in familial ALS?** | The gene encodes for superoxide dismutase (see Table 48–1, G). |
| **What is the overall incidence of ALS?** | 1 per 100,000 in the United States |
| **What is the typical age of onset?** | After 50 years of age, it increases progressively. |
| **Are there known risk factors for developing sporadic ALS?** | No |
| **What anatomic areas are affected in ALS?** | Lateral corticospinal tracts, corticobulbar tracts, and lower motor neurons (LMNs) without involvement of sensory pathways |
| **What are the characteristic physical findings in ALS?** | Combination of upper motor neuron (UMN) and LMN signs |

**What is a UMN?**

A nerve cell body in the primary motor cortex as well as its axon (before it synapses with a cranial or spinal LMN)

**What is an LMN?**

A nerve cell body in a cranial motor nucleus or the anterior horn of the spinal cord and its axon in a cranial or somatic peripheral nerve, which supplies motor fibers to muscles

**What are five signs of UMN lesions?**

1. Hyperreflexia
2. Spasticity
3. Extensor plantar responses (Babinski's sign)
4. Clonus
5. Weakness

**What are five signs of LMN lesions?**

1. Hyporeflexia
2. Flaccidity
3. Atrophy
4. Fasciculations
5. Weakness

**What is spasticity?**

Increased muscle tone with resistance to passive stretch during the initial phase of excursion; there may then be an abrupt decrease in resistance (the so-called clasp-knife phenomenon)

**What are fasciculations?**

Irregular contractions of muscle fibers that appear as ripples under the skin and indicate the irregular spontaneous firing of motor units; they may be caused by a variety of factors

**What do fasciculations indicate in a patient with ALS?**

They indicate dying anterior horn or cranial nerve motor nuclei.

**Are fasciculations without weakness a sign of ALS?**

No—many otherwise healthy persons experience benign fasciculations

**Which otherwise healthy persons are especially prone to seek medical consultation for muscle fasciculations?**

Medical personnel

**What factors predispose otherwise healthy people to fasciculations?**

Fatigue, cold, anxiety, recent exercise

**What motor functions are virtually always spared in ALS?**

Bowel and bladder continence

**Why?**

ALS is a disease of the somatic (voluntary) motor, not the autonomic, nervous system

**What are the sensory findings in ALS?**

Normal

**What are the characteristic EMG findings?**

Widespread denervation and reinnervation

**What is the natural history of ALS?**

Inexorable progression, with death in 3–5 years secondary to aspiration pneumonia or ventilatory failure

**What relatively common condition in the elderly can produce UMN and LMN deficits and mimic ALS?**

Cervical spondylosis

**What is another disease of the cervical spinal cord that can mimic ALS?**

Syringomyelia

**What three signs help distinguish ALS from cervical spinal cord diseases?**

Tongue fasciculations, brisk jaw jerk, and spastic dysarthria in ALS

# 24

# Multiple Sclerosis

| | |
|---|---|
| **What category of disease is multiple sclerosis (MS)?** | Demyelinating |
| **What cell makes CNS myelin?** | Oligodendroglia |
| **What cell makes peripheral nervous system (PNS) myelin?** | Schwann cells |
| **Does MS involve the PNS?** | No |
| **What age group is at greatest risk of a first attack of MS?** | Young adults |
| **What is the association of MS with geography?** | Individuals who spent their childhood in cool climates are at increased risk. |
| **What are some current theories about the etiology of MS?** | Genetic susceptibility<br>CNS immunity altered possibly by environmental agent, perhaps a virus<br>Oligodendroglial membranes are target of immune attack |
| **What two features are needed to clinically diagnose MS?** | Exacerbations and remissions<br>Lesions in more than one area of CNS |
| **Define exacerbation.** | Loss or deterioration of a neurologic function |
| **Define remission.** | Return to or toward normal function |
| **What is the most common course?** | Relapsing–remitting |
| **How do most MS patients accumulate neurologic deficits?** | Some of their remissions are incomplete due to irreparable axonal damage. |

| | |
|---|---|
| **What are the signs and symptoms of MS?** | Any symptom/sign appropriate to a lesion in CNS white matter. Rarely gray matter signs, such as seizures and altered mental state, occur. |
| **What specific symptoms are most common?** | Paresthesias<br>Blurred or double vision<br>Incoordination<br>Urinary urgency and/or incontinence |
| **What is Devic's disease?** | Optic neuritis and transverse myelitis |

## EYE PROBLEMS IN MS

### OPTIC NEURITIS

| | |
|---|---|
| **What is optic neuritis?** | Inflammatory demyelination of the optic nerve |
| **Is it frequent in MS?** | Yes, but MS is not the only cause. |
| **What are two symptoms of optic neuritis?** | Blurred vision and pain on eye movement |
| **Characterize the visual acuity.** | Reduced |
| **Will refraction help acuity in optic neuritis?** | No |
| **What is the appearance of the optic disc in optic neuritis?** | Pink, swollen with indistinct margin if papilla is involved; normal, if involvement is retrobulbar. |
| **What pupillary abnormality occurs in optic neuritis?** | An afferent pupillary defect |
| **What is it?** | Reduced pupilloconstriction on ipsilateral eye illumination but with constriction on contralateral illumination |
| **What is the papilla?** | The optic nerve head in the retina |
| **What is the name for optic neuritis behind the optic nerve head?** | Retrobulbar neuritis |

| | |
|---|---|
| **What phrase describes the funduscopic appearance of retrobulbar neuritis?** | It is normal: "The patient sees nothing and the doctor also sees nothing." |
| **What is the appearance of the optic disc in optic atrophy?** | Pallor, especially temporal area; distinct disc margin |
| **What visual field defect is common in optic neuritis or atrophy?** | A central scotoma |
| **What is a scotoma?** | An island of blindness in a sea of vision |
| **Name a funduscopic examination finding, resulting from previous optic neuritis?** | Optic atrophy |

## INTERNUCLEAR OPHTHALMOPLEGIA (INO)

| | |
|---|---|
| **What is INO?** | Inability to adduct the eye with voluntary lateral gaze, but with preservation of adduction on convergence |
| **What causes INO?** | A lesion, often demyelinative, in the medial longitudinal fasciculus (MLF) |
| **What two paths run through the MLF?** | Connections to the contralateral CN III nucleus from (1) the pontine lateral gaze center near CN VI nucleus and (2) from the vestibular system |
| **What other sign usually accompanies the gaze palsy?** | Nystagmus |
| **Why can the eyes adduct on convergence, but not on lateral gaze?** | The convergence path does not run in the MLF. |
| **What is the path for eye convergence?** | Retina to tectum of the midbrain (via the optic nerve, chiasm, tract, and lateral geniculate) to midbrain nuclei, then to *bilateral* CN III nuclei |

## COMMON CLINICAL FINDINGS IN MS

| | |
|---|---|
| **What is Lhermitte's sign?** | An electric sensation descending the vertebrae with neck flexion |
| **In addition to MS, what is another cause?** | Cervical stenosis or other mechanical irritation to posterior columns |
| **What are girdle paresthesias in MS?** | Pressure sensation hugging the trunk |
| **What excretory problems are frequent in spinal MS?** | Urinary urgency and incontinence<br>Urinary hesitancy<br>Constipation |
| **What is the usual bladder dysfunction in MS?** | Urinary sphincter dyssynergia |
| **What is urinary sphincter dyssynergia?** | Simultaneous contraction of the urinary bladder detrusor smooth muscle and the voluntary muscles of the pelvic floor |
| **What is MS fatigue?** | Midday loss of energy unrelated to other MS signs or symptoms |
| **What is heat sensitivity in MS?** | Transient presence of a neurologic deficit or symptom accompanying increased body temperature |
| **What is the prevalence of seizures in MS?** | Approximately 5% |
| **What is Uhtoff's sign?** | Transient neurologic deficit when hot |

## DIAGNOSIS

| | |
|---|---|
| **What are the two most helpful paraclinical tests to diagnose MS?** | MRI and evaluation of CSF |
| **Characterize MRI findings in a patient with MS.** | Multifocal areas of increased intensity on T2 (and proton density) images in the CNS white matter |
| **What is another common cause for these lesions on MRI?** | Small scattered subcortical ischemic infarcts |

| | |
|---|---|
| **What is the classic location of MS lesions on MRI?** | Periventricular, especially in corpus callosum (see Chapter 43, Exercise 5) |
| **What are Dawson's fingers?** | Periventricular MS lesions on MRI at right angles to the ependyma |
| **Which CSF finding is most specific for MS?** | Presence of unique oligoclonal bands |
| **What are oligoclonal bands?** | Monoclonal bands of intrathecally synthesized IgG on immune focused CSF electrophoresis |
| **Are these oligoclonal bands present in blood?** | No—they are unique to the CSF |
| **What CSF changes are consistent with a recent MS exacerbation?** | Elevated WBCs (usually < 50 lymphocytes)<br>Elevated myelin basic protein |
| **What CSF changes persist between exacerbations?** | Presence of oligoclonal bands<br>Increased rate of globulin synthesis |

## DRUG THERAPY IN MS

| | |
|---|---|
| **Is there a cure or prevention of MS?** | No |
| **What is the role of steroids?** | They will often shorten an exacerbation. |
| **What four drugs are available for immunomodulation of MS?** | Interferon-$\beta$ (Betaseron, Avonex, and Rebif) and glatiramer (Copaxone) |
| **What is the role of interferon-$\beta$ and glatiramer?** | Reduces exacerbation rate by about 33% |
| **In which clinical course of MS is interferon-$\beta$ or glatiramer most helpful?** | Relapsing–remitting |
| **Name three other drugs sometimes used in MS that is worsening.** | Mitoxantrone (Novantrone), cyclosporin, and methotrexate |

| | |
|---|---|
| **Name three drugs used to reduce MS fatigue.** | Amantadine (Symmetrel), modafinil (Provigil), and methylphenidate (Ritalin) |
| **Name four drugs used to reduce spasticity in MS.** | Baclofen (Lioresal), tizanidine (Zanaflex), dantrolene (Dantrium), and benzodiazepines |
| **Name three drugs used to reduce paresthesias in MS.** | Amitriptyline, gabapentin (Neurontin), and carbamazepine |
| **Name two drugs used for urinary urge incontinence.** | Oxybutynin (Ditropan) and tolterodine (Detrol) |

## ACUTE DISSEMINATED ENCEPHALOMYELITIS (ADEM)

| | |
|---|---|
| **Are MS and ADEM the same?** | Unknown |
| **What class of disease are they?** | Demyelinating |
| **Which best mimics the animal model, experimental allergic encephalomyelitis?** | ADEM |
| **Which is more likely to commence in childhood?** | ADEM |
| **Which is more likely to follow a specific insult: viral illness, immunization, or insect sting?** | ADEM |
| **Which is more likely a one time event?** | ADEM |
| **Are any of these distinctions absolute?** | No |

# 25

# Acute Intermittent Porphyria

## BASIC CONSIDERATIONS

| | |
|---|---|
| **What are the two classes of porphyria?** | Hepatic and erythropoietic |
| **Which class affects the nervous system?** | Hepatic |
| **What are the two types of hepatic porphyria?** | Acute intermittent porphyria (AIP) and variegate porphyria |
| **Which type of hepatic porphyria is most commonly seen in the United States?** | AIP |

## AIP

| | |
|---|---|
| **How is AIP transmitted?** | Genetically, as an autosomal dominant trait |
| **AIP is a defect in the production of what substance?** | Heme |
| **Is AIP associated with cutaneous sensitivity?** | No |
| **What three groups of substances can induce an attack of AIP?** | Alcohol, some prescription drugs, and estrogen |
| **What anticonvulsant classically induces an attack?** | Barbiturates, but so can other anticonvulsants |
| **Why do certain drugs produce an acute attack?** | Because they induce aminolevulinic acid (ALA) synthease |

| | |
|---|---|
| **What are three symptoms of an acute attack?** | 1. Abdominal pain<br>2. Psychosis or other encephalopathy<br>3. Seizures |
| **Can AIP affect both the central and peripheral nervous systems?** | Yes |
| **Name two examples of a CNS effect.** | 1. Seizures<br>2. Encephalopathy |
| **Name one example of PNS effect.** | Subacute motor neuropathy (primarily axonal) |
| **How do deep tendon reflex abnormalities differ from the findings in other neuropathies?** | Reflexes are diminished or absent, but paradoxically ankle jerks may be maintained |
| **Can AIP affect the autonomic nervous system?** | Yes |
| **Name two examples of an autonomic effect.** | 1. Hypertension<br>2. Tachycardia |
| **In an acute attack of AIP, what two substances are elevated in the urine (and thus useful for diagnosis)?** | ALA and porphobilinogen |
| **What is a characteristic feature of urine in AIP?** | Darkens (turns orange-brown) on standing |
| **What is the treatment of an acute attack?** | IV hematin and glucose to inhibit ALA synthesis, and $\beta$-blockers to treat hypertension and tachycardia |

## VARIEGATE PORPHYRIA

| | |
|---|---|
| **What is a distinguishing symptom of variegate porphyria?** | Cutaneous sensitivity to sunlight |
| **In what geographic area does variegate porphyria occur?** | South Africa |

# 26

## Central Pontine Myelinolysis

| | |
|---|---|
| **What is central pontine myelinolysis (CPM)?** | Demyelination of white matter in the base of the pons |
| **Name two types of patients most susceptible to CPM.** | Alcoholics with poor nutrition<br>Persons taking thiazide diuretics who lose sodium in urine |
| **What is the electrolyte abnormality and clinical scenario in which a patient develops CPM?** | Rapid intravenous correction of hyponatremia |
| **What is the typical clinical course of a patient who develops CPM?** | Shortly after electrolyte correction, the patient feels better, then becomes confused. |
| **What are the neurologic and physical findings in CPM?** | Mental changes (either obtundation or coma) and spastic tetraparesis; the ability to chew, talk, or swallow may also be impaired |
| **Which imaging test should be ordered, MRI or CT?** | MRI |
| **Why?** | On CT, the dense bones in the base of the skull cause scatter artifact to distort the clarity of pontine image. |
| **How should hyponatremia be corrected so that CPM is avoided?** | Use normal saline, infuse slowly, and check sodium levels every 2–3 hours |
| **How rapidly may serum sodium safely rise?** | No faster than 0.5 mEq/L/hr |

# 27

# Ménière's Disease

**What is the clinical triad of symptoms of Ménière's disease?**

Tinnitus, deafness, and vertigo

**What is the etiology of this disease?**

Unknown

**What is the pathology?**

Labyrinthine hydrops

**What is labyrinthine hydrops?**

Distention of the endolymphatic system of the labyrinth caused by excess endolymphatic fluid

**Describe the tinnitus in Ménière's disease.**

Either pulsatile or constant sound; usually in only one (the affected) ear

**Describe the deafness.**

Initially intermittent; eventually constant sensorineural hearing loss occurs

**Do hearing aids help?**

Not usually, because there is poor neural conduction

**Is the deafness usually unilateral or bilateral?**

Unilateral in 90% of patients

**Describe the vertigo.**

Rotational, often with autonomic accompaniments of nausea, vomiting, or sense of flushing

**Name two common activities likely to initiate the vertigo.**

1. Turning over in bed
2. Rotating the head (e.g., as done when driving or stepping off the curb to cross the street)

**Does closing one's eyes help the vertigo?**

No, it persists.

**Are tinnitus and deafness most indicative of central or peripheral disease?**

Peripheral—usually the cochlea, although can be of eighth cranial nerve etiology

**Which is the most disabling manifestation?**

Vertigo. It is usually episodic and disappears with time, whereas the deafness and tinnitus are lifelong.

**Is there effective, curative therapy?**

No, but surgical decompression of the endolymphatic system may be attempted.

**What three types of drugs may provide symptomatic relief?**

**Motion sickness medications** (e.g., meclizine) and **sedatives** (e.g., diazepam) help vertigo, and **diuretics** (e.g., acetazolamide) may relieve endolymphatic fluid excess.

# Benign Paroxysmal Positional Vertigo

| | |
|---|---|
| **How is benign paroxysmal positional vertigo (BPPV) different from Ménière's disease?** | In BPPV, there is neither tinnitus nor deafness. |
| **Describe the vertigo in BPPV.** | Rotational vertigo commences several seconds after a head turn. It usually lasts for 15–45 seconds and may occur several times a day. |
| **What is a common bedside diagnostic test?** | The Hallpike maneuver |
| **Describe it.** | The sitting patient quickly lies supine and drops his head 30° down and over the end of the examining table. Lateral rotation of the head stimulates the semicircular canal endolymph and, after a brief latency, initiates short-lived vertigo. |
| **What is the etiology of BPPV?** | Uncertain—perhaps dislocation of labyrinthine otoliths secondary to head trauma or sludging of endolymph |
| **What is a nondrug therapy?** | Frequent daily exercises that elicit vertigo and eventually fatigue the BPPV or redistribute sludged endolymph |
| **What are some drug therapies?** | Meclizine, an anti–motion sickness medication<br>Diazepam |

# Neurologic Complications of Systemic Illnesses

## CANCER

| | |
|---|---|
| **In what five ways may metastases to the nervous system present?** | 1. Progressive focal neurological deficit<br>2. Seizures<br>3. Headache<br>4. Increased ICP<br>5. Mental status change |
| **What are two neurologic complications of nonsurgical cancer treatment?** | Chemotherapeutic agents may cause peripheral neuropathy; radiation may cause necrosis of brain. |
| **What are the paraneoplastic syndromes that may affect each level of the nervous system, going from muscle to brain?** | |
| **Muscle?** | Dermatomyositis, polymyositis |
| **Neuromuscular junction?** | Lambert-Eaton myasthenic syndrome |
| **Peripheral nerve?** | Peripheral neuropathy (sensory or mixed) |
| **Spinal cord?** | Myelopathy |
| **Brain?** | Leukoencephalopathy, "limbic" encephalitis |

## DIABETES

| | |
|---|---|
| **Which part of the nervous system is most frequently affected in diabetes?** | Peripheral nerves |

**What pathologic process in diabetes damages the peripheral nerves?**

Ischemic infarction

**Name four different forms of diabetic neuropathy by localization.**

1. Mononeuropathy
2. Polyneuropathy
3. Plexopathy
4. Mononeuropathy multiplex

**Can diabetes involve both motor and sensory fibers?**

Yes

**Which form of diabetic neuropathy is most common?**

Distal, primarily sensory, polyneuropathy

**What are common symptoms of diabetic sensory polyneuropathy?**

Pain, tingling, burning, numbness

**What are the typical anatomic locations for these symptoms?**

Hands and feet

**What jargon term describes this location?**

Stocking–glove distribution

**What are the distribution and pattern for stocking–glove neuropathy?**

Distal, symmetrical, graded sensory loss

**What is the most common reflex abnormality on motor exam?**

Bilaterally absent Achilles reflexes

**Other than discomfort, what is the major morbidity to the patient with sensory neuropathy?**

Failure to perceive pain, resulting in ulcers, trauma, infection, and burns

**What is the best laboratory test to diagnose diabetic neuropathy?**

Nerve conduction velocity (NCV) study

| | |
|---|---|
| **Name a situation in which slowed NCV is not seen in diabetic sensory neuropathy?** | Small fiber neuropathy with major symptoms of pain and burning instead of numbness |
| **Name three drugs that help alleviate the symptoms.** | 1. Tricyclics<br>2. Anticonvulsants, including gabapentin (Neurontin)<br>3. Capsaicin |
| **What is capsaicin?** | A centrally acting depleter of substance P |
| **What is the term used to describe diabetes affecting a single nerve instead of multiple nerves?** | Diabetic mononeuropathy |
| **Which nerves can be affected by diabetic mononeuropathy?** | Cranial nerves, especially CN III and VI<br>Spinal roots<br>Single peripheral nerves, such as the sciatic, radial, or femoral nerves |
| **In a diabetic third-nerve palsy, why may the pupil be spared?** | Parasympathetic pupillary fibers are on the outside of the nerve and retain their blood supply, even when the core of the nerve infarcts from disease of small penetrating vessels. |
| **What is the main differential diagnosis of diabetic third-nerve palsy?** | Posterior communicating artery aneurysm with third-nerve compression |
| **Describe the pupil in third-nerve compression?** | Dilated |

## THYROID DISORDERS

### HYPERTHYROIDISM

| | |
|---|---|
| **What are four neurologic complications of hyperthyroidism?** | 1. Tremor (due to adrenergic excess)<br>2. Weakness<br>3. Eye signs (e.g., exophthalmos, lid lag, and convergence weakness)<br>4. Emotional lability |

| | |
|---|---|
| **What lab result is most likely to establish the diagnosis?** | Decreased thyroid-stimulating hormone (TSH) |
| **Which hyperthyroid manifestation may not be associated with low TSH?** | Graves' eye disease (exophthalmic goiter) |
| **Name three daily activities in which the muscle weakness of hyperthyroidism often first appears.** | 1. Climbing stairs<br>2. Combing hair<br>3. Arising from a chair |
| **What are four signs of hyperthyroid infiltrative ophthalmopathy?** | 1. Exophthalmos<br>2. Ophthalmoplegia<br>3. Chemosis<br>4. Optic atrophy (if severe) |
| **What two hyperthyroid eye signs are due to adrenergic excess rather than infiltration?** | Lid lag on down gaze, lid retraction |
| **What immune-mediated neurologic disease may be associated with autoimmune hyperthyroidism?** | Myasthenia gravis |

## HYPOTHYROIDISM

| | |
|---|---|
| **What are three neurologic manifestations of hypothyroidism?** | 1. Myopathy<br>2. Neuropathy<br>3. Encephalopathy |
| **Characterize the tendon stretch reflex in patients with hypothyroidism.** | Delayed relaxation (a nonspecific finding) |
| **Can both hypo- and hyperthyroidism cause weakness?** | Yes |
| **What are two mechanisms of weakness in hypothyroidism?** | Myopathy and peripheral neuropathy |

| | |
|---|---|
| **What does a positive Tinel's sign at the wrist in a patient with hypothyroidism suggest?** | Compression neuropathy of the median nerve in the carpal tunnel (i.e., carpal tunnel syndrome) due to mucopolysaccharide deposition |
| **What is the definition of myxedema?** | Generally speaking, it is the clinical picture of hypothyroidism. Specifically, it is subcutaneous deposition of mucinous (myxo-) material, resulting in nonpitting edema. |
| **Describe myoedema.** | Visible local swelling upon tapping a hypothyroid muscle |
| **What is myxedema madness?** | Hypothyroid psychosis |
| **What are two reversible cognitive abnormalities in hypothyroid encephalopathy?** | Mental dullness and memory impairment |

## NUTRITIONAL DEFICIENCIES (SEE CHAPTER 16, ALCOHOL AND THE NERVOUS SYSTEM)

| | |
|---|---|
| **What nutritional state predisposes a person to Wernicke-Korsakoff syndrome?** | Malnutrition, especially in alcoholics |
| **Deficiency of what vitamin is responsible for most signs of Wernicke-Korsakoff syndrome?** | Thiamine (vitamin $B_1$) |
| **What is the common medical term for multinutritional polyneuropathy?** | Beri-beri |
| **Which persons in the United States are at highest risk for developing beri-beri?** | Alcoholics |

| | |
|---|---|
| **What is the term for beri-beri with neurologic symptoms?** | "Dry" beri-beri (cardiac symptoms are "wet" beri-beri) |
| **What is combined systems disease?** | Degeneration of the posterior and lateral columns of the spinal cord |
| **Deficiency of what vitamin is causative?** | Cyanocobalamin (vitamin $B_{12}$) |
| **What vitamin deficiency causes night blindness?** | Vitamin A |
| **When ingested in excess, what vitamin can cause pseudotumor cerebri?** | Vitamin A |
| **What neurologic condition may result from excess pyridoxine?** | Sensory peripheral neuropathy |
| **Isoniazid peripheral neuropathy is associated with what vitamin deficiency?** | Pyridoxine |
| **What substance must be present for gut absorption of vitamin $B_{12}$?** | Intrinsic factor made by parietal cells in the stomach |
| **Too-rapid repletion of hyponatremia can cause what neurologic condition?** | Central pontine myelinolysis |
| **What nutritional deficiency causes pellagra?** | Niacin |
| **What is the classic clinical triad of pellagra?** | The three D's:<br>1. Diarrhea<br>2. Dermatitis<br>3. Dementia |

## NUTRITIONAL DEFICIENCY IN INFANCY AND CHILDHOOD

**What is the fetal consequence of severe maternal iodine deficiency during pregnancy?**

Cretinism

**An infant has a seizure after 1 week of being fed formula that is diluted 75% with water. What blood chemistry abnormalities should be sought?**

Hyponatremia
Hypoglycemia
Hypocalcemia
Hypomagnesemia

**What vitamin deficiency can cause infantile seizures?**

Pyridoxine

**What is kwashiorkor?**

Profound dietary protein deficiency in childhood

**Deficiency of what maternal vitamin contributes to fetal neural tube anomalies?**

Folic acid

## TOXINS AND THE NERVOUS SYSTEM

**What are the three most common syndromes that occur following acute carbon monoxide poisoning?**

1. Dementia
2. Parkinsonism
3. Cerebellar ataxia

**What is the skin color of a person who died from carbon monoxide poisoning?**

Cherry red

**What color is the brain, and why?**

It is red also, due to carboxy hemoglobin.

**What does lead intoxication produce in adults?**

Axonal peripheral neuropathy

**What does lead intoxication produce in children?**

Encephalopathy, beginning with personality change and irritability, leading to seizures and coma; due to brain swelling and increased ICP

**What are the most common signs of manganese intoxication?**

Akinesia, rigidity and dystonia; due to damage to the globus pallidus and subthalamic nucleus

**What are the CNS effects of arsenic poisoning?**

Encephalopathy, peripheral neuropathy

**What is the dermatologic sign of chronic arsenic intoxication?**

White transverse bands across the nails (Mees' lines)

**Organophosphorus insecticides are acetylcholinesterase inhibitors. What are the clinical signs of acute organophosphorus poisoning?**

Bradycardia
Hypotension
Sweating
Weakness, leading to respiratory failure
Ataxia
Confusion

**What illicit drug can produce parkinsonism within 1 week of injection?**

MPTP (1-methyl-4-phenyl-tetrahydropyridine), which is a compound that could contaminate meperidine or heroin sold on the street. It is toxic to CNS dopamine neurons and produces dose-related parkinsonism.

**What movement disorder could be caused by chronic amphetamine or cocaine abuse?**

Quick involuntary muscle jerks, such as chorea or tics

**What is a neurologic complication of cocaine use?**

Seizures

# 30

# Neurologic Complications of Anesthesia and Surgery

## BASIC CONSIDERATIONS

**Do most postsurgical neurologic complications involve the peripheral or central nervous system?**

Peripheral nervous system

**Are most postsurgical peripheral neurologic complications caused by anesthetic drugs?**

No, the majority are unrelated to the anesthesia itself. Most are due to positioning.

**What CNS dysfunction is common in the elderly following general anesthesia?**

Temporary postoperative confusion is common. Prolonged or permanent changes (e.g., in memory or cognition) are rare.

**What is the incidence of perioperative stroke?**

Following non-neurologic, non-cardiac surgery, the incidence is rare (less than 1 in 2500). Following carotid or cardiopulmonary surgery, the incidence is associated with the experience of the surgical team and may range from 0.2% to 20%.

**What is the etiology of perioperative stroke?**

Most are thrombotic and embolic (primarily cardiac), rather than hypotensive or hemorrhagic.

**What are five neurologic complications following spinal or epidural anesthesia?**

1. Postdural puncture headache (PDPH)
2. Direct needle trauma
3. Epidural hematoma
4. Aseptic or infectious meningitis
5. Anterior spinal artery thrombosis

| | |
|---|---|
| **What is the etiology of backache following spinal/epidural anesthesia?** | Usually, ligament strain associated with back muscle relaxation and surgical positioning; must also consider rare but more serious causes, such as epidural abscess or epidural hematoma |

## PDPH (See also Chapter 6, Headache, Chapter 44, LP)

| | |
|---|---|
| **What are two vernacular names for PDPH?** | Post LP headache and "spinal headache" |
| **How common is PDPH in spinal anesthesia?** | Less than 3% of spinal anesthetics |
| **What is the etiology of PDPH?** | Persistent leak of CSF through dural puncture, resulting in decreased ICP |
| **What are the characteristics of a PDPH?** | Onset 1–2 days after dural puncture<br>Bilateral<br>Worse when patient is erect, better when supine<br>More common in young women<br>More common following use of large-gauge spinal needle |
| **Does remaining flat after LP reduce risk for PDPH?** | Unknown—but it is common practice to remain supine for a short duration after LP |
| **What is the treatment of PDPH?** | Initially, bed rest, hydration, analgesics, and caffeine are used. If the PDPH persists more than 24 hours, an epidural blood patch is used. |
| **How is a blood patch performed?** | Aseptic placement of 10-20 ml of autologous blood into the epidural space at the level of the dural puncture/CSF leak, often under fluoroscopy |
| **What is a home remedy using caffeine that sometimes works?** | Drink 2 liters of cola |

# POSTSURGICAL PERIPHERAL NERVE COMPLICATIONS

**What is the cause of peripheral nerve injury following anesthesia?**

Ischemia from nerve stretching or compression during anesthesia

**What are some surgery-related causes of peripheral nerve injury?**

Position of the unconscious patient on the table
Surgical retractions
Surgical trauma
Tourniquet pressure
Cast or dressing application

**What is the most common upper extremity nerve injury?**

Brachial plexus injury, primarily from abducting the arm greater than 90°

**What anatomical feature contributes to compressive ulnar nerve injury?**

Its superficial path along the medial aspect of the elbow

**What is the most common lower extremity nerve injury?**

The common peroneal nerve

**How does this injury occur?**

It results from compression between the fibula and a metal brace utilized for the lithotomy position.

**What is its most common neurologic presentation?**

Foot drop

**What are two neurologic contraindications to use of the depolarizing muscle relaxant succinylcholine?**

1. Neuromuscular diseases (e.g., muscular dystrophy)
2. Denervating injuries (e.g., spinal cord injury)

**Why is succinylcholine contraindicated in neuromuscular and denervating disorders?**

Life-threatening hyperkalemia caused by release of potassium by denervated muscle

**What neuromuscular disease may prolong the paralyzing effects of nondepolarizing muscle relaxants, such as vecuronium?**

Myasthenia gravis and myasthenic syndromes

**Why?**

Vecuronium paralyzes muscle by blocking acetylcholine receptors, which are already abnormal in myasthenia gravis

# 31 Drugs and the Nervous System

## MECHANISMS OF NEUROACTIVE DRUGS

| | |
|---|---|
| **Name six neurotransmitter systems commonly affected by drugs.** | 1. Glutamate<br>2. $\gamma$-Aminobutyric acid (GABA)<br>3. Serotonin<br>4. Acetylcholine (ACh)<br>5. Epinephrine (adrenaline)<br>6. Dopamine |
| **Do some drugs affect more than one system?** | Yes |
| **What is an *agonist* drug?** | Generally (and for this book), this term refers to any drug that enhances transmission in a specific neurotransmitter system. In strict pharmacologic usage, this term describes a drug that binds at the exact same site as the natural neurotransmitter. |
| **What is an *antagonist* drug?** | Generally speaking, it is a drug that has the opposite effect of an agonist drug. |

## GLUTAMATE

| | |
|---|---|
| **Why is glutamate neurotransmission important?** | 1. Glutamate is the most common excitatory neurotransmitter.<br>2. Activation of the NMDA subtype of glutamate receptor may be important in cell death, via elevated intracellular $Ca^{2+}$, during status epilepticus and other conditions. |
| **What specific NMDA antagonists are approved in the United States?** | None. Ketamine is a nonspecific NMDA antagonist but is only used in general anesthesia. MK801 has been studied for use in epilepsy, but it is not available. |

## GABA

| | |
|---|---|
| **What is the role of GABA in normal neurotransmission?** | It is an inhibitory neurotransmitter. |
| **Name two types of drugs used to treat seizures that are GABA agonists (i.e., they enhance GABA transmission).** | 1. Barbiturates<br>2. Benzodiazepines |
| **What is a neurologic side effect of activating the GABA system?** | Sedation |
| **Name a benzodiazepine antagonist (i.e., a drug that inhibits the GABA system) used to reverse the effects of benzodiazepines.** | Flumazenil |
| **What is a neurologic side effect of inhibiting the GABA system?** | Seizures |
| **What is the neurologic risk of withdrawal of benzodiazepines?** | Acute benzodiazepine withdrawal seizures |

## SEROTONIN

| | |
|---|---|
| **What serotonin (5HT) agonists are used to treat migraines?** | Triptans, such as sumatriptan, are agonists at the 5HT-1 receptor. |
| **What class of drugs that activates the serotonin system is used to treat depression?** | Selective serotonin reuptake inhibitors (SSRIs), such as fluoxetine (Prozac) and sertraline (Zoloft) |

## ACh

| | |
|---|---|
| **What two drugs that enhance transmission in the ACh system are used in myasthenia gravis?** | 1. Pyridostigmine (Mestinon)<br>2. Edrophonium (Tensilon) |

| | |
|---|---|
| **How is the mechanism of action of these drugs different from direct-acting ACh-agonist drugs?** | They are anticholinesterase drugs, which inhibit breakdown of ACh rather than activate ACh receptors directly. |
| **What are three side effects of Tensilon administration during a Tensilon test?** | Bradycardia, nausea, perspiration |
| **What anticholinesterase drugs are used to treat dementia?** | Tacrine (Cognex), donepezil (Aricept), rivastigmine (Exelon), galantamine (Reminyl) |
| **Name two ACh antagonists used to treat motion sickness and glaucoma.** | 1. Scopolamine<br>2. Atropine |
| **Name two drugs, primarily used for their anticholinergic effects, that are used to treat parkinsonism.** | 1. Benztropine (Cogentin)<br>2. Trihexyphenidyl (Artane) |
| **What are two systemic side effects of ACh blockade?** | Dry mouth, blurry vision |

## EPINEPHRINE

| | |
|---|---|
| **Name two adrenergic agonists.** | Epinephrine, pseudoephedrine |
| **What are two systemic side effects of activating the adrenergic system?** | Tachycardia, hypertension |
| **Name an illicit drug that is an adrenergic agonist?** | Cocaine |
| **How does it act?** | Inhibits epinephrine reuptake |

## DOPAMINE (See Chapter 11)

| | |
|---|---|
| **What drugs best treat Parkinson's disease?** | Dopamine agonists and levodopa carbidopa |

| | |
|---|---|
| **What are two neurologic side effects of dopaminergic activation?** | Psychosis, dyskinesia |
| **Name a class of drugs with primary antidopaminergic effects.** | Neuroleptic antipsychotics |
| **What are three movement disorders caused by neuroleptics?** | 1. Parkinsonism (i.e., rigidity, resting tremor, and bradykinesia)<br>2. Akathisia<br>3. Tardive dyskinesia |
| **What are two classes of drugs used to treat psychiatric disorders that have anticholinergic and antiadrenergic effects?** | Tricyclic antidepressants, neuroleptic antipsychotics |
| **What class of drugs has antidopaminergic, anticholinergic, and antiadrenergic effects?** | Neuroleptic antipsychotics |
| **What aminergic functions are responsible for the three most common neurologic side effects of these drugs?** | Antidopaminergic effects cause parkinsonism.<br>Anticholinergic effects cause dry mouth and blurry vision (impaired accommodation).<br>Antiadrenergic effects cause orthostatic hypotension. |
| **How can metoclopramide (Reglan) affect the nervous system?** | Because it is a moderately potent dopamine antagonist, metoclopramide can cause parkinsonism or tardive dyskinesia. |
| **What is tardive dyskinesia?** | A delayed hyperkinetic movement disorder arising late in the course of treatment with neuroleptic (antipsychotic) drugs. |
| **What are the most common features of tardive dyskinesia?** | Repetitive lip puckering, mouth opening, and tongue protrusion; younger patients are more likely to develop choreoathetotic limb movements than are older patients. |

| | |
|---|---|
| **What is an oculogyric crisis?** | An acute dystonia (i.e., sustained, involuntary muscle contraction) of ocular, face, and neck muscles that occurs during a treatment course with neuroleptics. |
| **When does an oculogyric crisis occur?** | Within a few days of initiating neuroleptics |

### Neuroleptic Malignant Syndrome (NMS)

| | |
|---|---|
| **What are the signs of NMS?** | Fever, depressed consciousness, rigidity, autonomic instability, elevated CPK |
| **What is the most serious result?** | Death |
| **What are two causes of NMS?** | 1. Use of dopamine-blocking (neuroleptic) drugs<br>2. Withdrawal from dopaminergic drugs in Parkinson's disease |

## NEUROLOGIC SIDE EFFECTS OF COMMON DRUGS

| | |
|---|---|
| **What is a serious neurologic side effect of overdosage with either tricyclic antidepressants or aminophylline/theophylline preparations?** | Refractory seizures |
| **What antidepressant has such a high risk of seizures in non-epileptics (0.4%) that it is contraindicated in epileptic patients?** | Bupropion (Wellbutrin) |
| **What is a common neurologic side effect of therapeutic lithium levels?** | Postural and intention tremor ("adrenergic tremor") |
| **Currently, what is the best treatment for this?** | Propranolol (Inderal) |
| **What are some neurologic side effects of IV amphetamine or cocaine abuse?** | Chorea, seizures, CNS vasculitis, stroke |

**What is a common neurologic side effect of treatment with cytosine arabinoside (AraC)?**

Cerebellar ataxia, which is usually reversible; it may be due to irreversible cerebellar degeneration

**How can vinca alkaloids (e.g., vincristine, vinblastine) affect the nervous system?**

By interfering with microtubule function and reducing axonal transport, they can cause peripheral neuropathy.

**How can chronic glucocorticoids (e.g., corticosteroid) affect muscle?**

They can cause mild, reversible proximal weakness (myopathy).

**How can high-dose methotrexate chemotherapy damage the nervous system?**

Methotrexate is a folic-acid antagonist and, in high doses, it can cause leukoencephalopathy and possibly seizures.

**What three drugs are associated with pseudotumor cerebri (benign intracranial hypertension)?**

1. Tetracyclines
2. Exogenous steroids
3. Vitamin A

**What are two potential neurologic side effects of exogenous estrogens?**

1. Exacerbation and/or precipitation of migraine
2. Stroke

**What is a serious neurologic side effect of toxic lidocaine levels?**

Seizures; sedation and agitation may occur, but are less serious

**What is the most common neurotoxic side effect of aminoglycoside antibiotics?**

Ototoxicity manifest as tinnitus, hearing loss, or vertigo

**What is the major neurotoxic side effect of high-dose penicillin?**

Generalized seizures and myoclonus, especially in patients with renal insufficiency

**What drug is routinely administered to prevent isoniazid (INH) neuropathy?**

Pyridoxine (Vitamin $B_6$)—50 mg/day

**What are the signs of sensory neuropathy due to megadoses (>2 g/day) of vitamin $B_6$ (pyridoxine)?**

Distal sensory loss in the legs and arms, decreased deep tendon reflexes, and sensory ataxia, but all with normal strength

**What is the role of folic acid in pregnancy?**

Maternal supplementation reduces fetal neural tube birth defects.

# 32 Neurologic Aspects of Bioterrorism

**Identify five clinical presentations consistent with exposure to an agent intended to injure many people.**

1. Acute respiratory distress
2. Acute rash with fever
3. Flu-like illness
4. Skin blistering
5. Neural (weakness, confusion)

**What is the best clinical clue to intended injury (bioterrorism)?**

Sudden occurrence of many similar patients

**Name two groups of dispersible agents affecting the nervous system.**

1. Neurotoxic chemical agents
2. Neurotoxic infectious agents

**How do *chemical* nerve agents work?**

They inhibit acetylcholinesterase

**What is the result?**

Excess ACh (parasympathomimetic)

**Describe the: pupils**
          **respiration**
          **G.I. tract**
          **muscles**
          **C.N.S.**

Miosis
Bronchospasm
Nausea, vomiting, diarrhea
Flaccid weakness; fasciculations
Confusion, coma, seizure, apnea, death

**Name two classes of *chemical nerve agents* of mass destruction.**

1. Carbamates, as in insecticides (Sevin)
2. Organophosphates (Sarin)

**Would these likely be "nerve gas"?**

More likely powder or liquid

**What *infectious agent* would cause mostly neurologic manifestations?**

Clostridium botulinum

**Is it a spore-forming bacterium?**

Yes, aids stability in dispersal

| | |
|---|---|
| **How does it affect the nervous system?** | Toxin inhibits ACh release at NMJ |
| **How does it clinically present?** | Progressive flaccid weakness |
| **Which muscles are affected first?** | Extraocular and pharyngeal usually |
| **Will there also be: mydriasis?** <br> **constipation?** <br> **dysphagia?** | Yes (with blurred vision) <br> Yes <br> Yes |
| **When would you suspect it?** | "Epidemic" GBS or Myasthenia Gravis |

# Section V

Pediatric Neurology

# 33

# Newborn Nursery Neurology

**Name two frequent neurologic abnormalities in newborns.**

1. Seizures
2. Hypotonia

**When should you suspect seizures in a newborn?**

Any repetitive motion, especially if it interrupts normal behavior

**Are these seizures easy to identify?**

No

**What best aids diagnosis?**

EEG

**What is the usual drug of choice for recurring seizures (epilepsy)?**

Phenobarbital

**What is the most common etiology?**

Hypoxic/ischemic encephalopathy

**What prenatal observation predicts it?**

Intrauterine fetal bradycardia

**Is the normal newborn hypotonic or hypertonic?**

Hypertonic

**Why?**

Incomplete myelinization of corticospinal tracts

**Cite three important causes of diffuse neonatal hypotonia.**

1. Perinatal hypoxia/ischemia
2. Maternal magnesium sulfate (tocolysis)
3. Maternal myasthenia gravis

**Which is most common?**

Hypoxic/ischemic encephalopathy

**List three common brain lesions causing neonatal hypotonia.**

1. Perinatal hypoxia-ischemia
2. Intracerebral hemorrhage
3. CNS infection

| | |
|---|---|
| **Is a neonate with weakness of *brain* origin alert to a normal degree?** | No |
| **State a cause of hypotonia in one arm.** | Brachial plexus injury at birth |
| **What is a neuromuscular junction cause of neonatal hypotonia and weakness?** | Transient neonatal myasthenia gravis |
| **How is it acquired?** | By antibody transmission from a mother with myasthenia gravis to the baby |
| **Can a normal awake baby see?** | Yes |
| **How do you test this?** | Put your face close to the baby's and watch him visually track as you move side to side. |
| **Will he root and suck?** | Yes |
| **Will he have normal labyrinthine function?** | Yes |
| **How do you test this?** | Hold awake baby and turn yourself in a circle. Baby will look ahead. |

# 34

# Hypotonia in Infancy: Age 1 to 6 Months

| | |
|---|---|
| **Define a "floppy infant."** | A hypotonic, weak infant |
| **Contrast the usual site of lesions causing hypotonia in adults versus children.** | Adults: Lower motor neuron<br>Children: Anywhere in the central or peripheral nervous system |
| **What are six levels (from proximal to distal) where disease can cause a floppy infant?** | 1. Brain<br>2. Spinal cord<br>3. Anterior horn cell<br>4. Peripheral nerve<br>5. Neuromuscular junction<br>6. Muscle |
| **Which is most common?** | Brain |
| **Name an anterior horn cell disease with infantile versus neonatal onset of hypotonic weakness.** | Spinal muscular atrophy or Werdnig-Hoffman disease |
| **What helps distinguish it from a brain etiology?** | Normal alertness |
| **Why is it an important diagnosis to make?** | It is fatal and transmitted by autosomal recessive inheritance. |
| **What infection that affects the neuromuscular junction causes a weak, hypotonic infant with a weak cry?** | Infantile botulism |
| **Name an accompanying condition.** | Constipation, usually |
| **Does Duchenne muscular dystrophy weakness commence in infancy?** | No. It presents in childhood. |

# 35

# Static Encephalopathy of Childhood

## CLINICAL CHARACTERISTICS

**Define static encephalopathy of childhood.**

Nonprogressive brain disorder with motor and/or intellectual deficits

**What is another commonly used term for the motor deficits?**

Cerebral palsy

**When does the onset of static encephalopathy usually occur?**

It is most often congenital, but acquired in the perinatal period (i.e., intrauterine, during delivery, or immediately following delivery). However, it may be acquired at any time of life.

**What three classes of etiology commonly cause static encephalopathy of childhood?**

1. Acquired insults
2. Developmental brain malformations
3. Chromosomal abnormalities

**Do metabolic disorders, such as mitochondrial diseases and organic and amino acidurias cause static or progressive encephalopathy?**

If untreated they are usually progressive, but when treatment is available, it may arrest progression (see Chapter 34).

**What two epileptic syndromes are associated with static encephalopathy of childhood?**

West's syndrome and Lennox-Gastaut syndrome (see Chapter 7)

**What features do both of these syndromes have in common?**

Static encephalopathy of childhood, intractable seizures, and characteristic EEG abnormalities

## ACQUIRED ETIOLOGIES

| | |
|---|---|
| **Is birth trauma the most common etiology of static encephalopathy?** | No. Intrauterine factors (i.e., genetic, prematurity, malformations, infections) are the most common causes. |
| **Using the mnemonic HHIIIM, characterize intrauterine brain injury.** | **H**ypoxic<br>**H**emorrhagic<br>**I**nfectious<br>**I**nherited<br>**I**schemic<br>**M**etabolic |
| **Using the mnemonic TORCH, list the causes of intrauterine brain infections.** | **T**oxoplasmosis<br>**O**ther (e.g., syphilis)<br>**R**ubella<br>**C**ytomegalovirus<br>**H**erpes simplex type II/HIV |
| **Which infants are at greatest risk of intraventricular hemorrhage?** | Premature births |
| **Where do such hemorrhages actually originate?** | Periventricular subependymal germinal matrix, not within the ventricle |
| **Grade, from 1 to 4, intraventricular hemorrhages of infancy based on the involved areas.** | Grade 1: germinal matrix, least severe<br>Grade 2: matrix and ventricle<br>Grade 3: grade 2 plus ventricular enlargement<br>Grade 4: grade 3 plus cortex, most severe |
| **What is the most common cause of static encephalopathy of childhood acquired after birth?** | Trauma |
| **What are watershed infarcts?** | Globally insufficient blood flow causing brain infarction of areas between major vascular territories |
| **What is a common cause of retinal hemorrhages and watershed infarcts in a baby?** | Shaken-baby syndrome (see Chapter 41) |

| | |
|---|---|
| **What is "shear injury" on MRI after head trauma?** | Microhemorrhages due to tearing of intraparenchymal arterioles and venules during deceleration. |
| **Using the mnemonic PAINT, characterize clinical manifestations of lead poisoning.** | **P**apilledema<br>**A**nemia<br>**I**ntermittent vomiting, include PICA<br>**N**europathy<br>**T**remors |
| **How do neurologic manifestations of lead poisoning differ in adults and children?** | In children they manifest as encephalopathy, whereas in adults they manifest as neuropathy. |
| **Characterize the RBCs in lead poisoning.** | Basophilic stippling |
| **Describe the features of a child with fetal alcohol syndrome.** | The child has small stature, head, and jaw as well as low weight and a thin upper lip. Epicanthal folds and short palpebral fissures are other features. |

**Table 35–1. Embryology and Malformations of the Brain and Spinal Cord**

| Developmental Day | Stage of Development | Associated CNS Malformation |
|---|---|---|
| Conception | | |
| Days 1–18 | Two-layered embryo | |
| Days 18–25 | Three-layered embryo<br>Formation of neural tube | Poor rostral fusion:<br>  encephalocele<br>Poor caudal fusion:<br>  meningomyelocele |
| Days 25–30 | Segmentation of intra-cranial neuraxis | Malformed subdivision into forebrain, midbrain, hindbrain |
| Days 30–45 | Rostral evagination and cleavage into mirror-image cerebral hemispheres | Failure: holoprosencephaly<br>  (arrhinencephaly) |
| Days 38–70 | Periventricular cellular proliferation, differentiation into neurons, and migration | Migration failures:<br>  lissencephaly, pachygyria,<br>  *polymicrogyria*, heterotopia |

A framework for understanding the relation between stages of embryonic development and congenital malformations of the nervous system

## DEVELOPMENTAL BRAIN MALFORMATIONS

Describe the following brain malformations:

| | |
|---|---|
| **Anencephaly** | Congenital absence of any brain substance above the brain stem |
| **Hydranencephaly** | Congenital absence of cerebral hemispheres with intact thalami and brain stem |
| **Lissencephaly** | Smooth brain lacking sulci, gyri, and normal six-layer cortex |
| **Hydrocephalus** | Dilated ventricles |
| **Schizencephaly** | A cleft in the brain, typically extending from the brain surface down to the ventricle |
| **Porencephaly** | A cystic cavity in the brain which may be congenital or acquired |

## CHROMOSOMAL ABNORMALITIES

| | |
|---|---|
| **What chromosome defect is the most common cause of mental retardation?** | Fragile X |
| **Describe the physical appearance of a person with fragile X syndrome.** | Long, narrow face; large ears; large testes |
| **What chromosome defect is the most common cause of Down's syndrome?** | Trisomy 21, which is the most common autosomal trisomy |
| **What neurologic disease is common in Down's syndrome patients after age 40?** | Alzheimer's disease |
| **What is cri du chat syndrome?** | A syndrome characterized by mental retardation, multiple congenital anomalies, and presence of a cat-like cry that is due to deletion of 5p |

**State the relation, if any, of maternal age at delivery and:**

    fragile X                  None

    **Down Syndrome**        Increased incidence in older mothers

# 36

# Neurocutaneous Disorders

| | |
|---|---|
| **What four diseases are classified as the *phakomatoses*, or neurocutaneous syndromes?** | 1. Neurofibromatosis<br>2. Tuberous sclerosis<br>3. von Hippel-Lindau disease<br>4. Sturge-Weber syndrome |
| **Which three are inherited?** | Neurofibromatosis, tuberous sclerosis, von Hippel-Lindau disease |
| **What organs are affected in the neurocutaneous disorders, and what common developmental origin do they share?** | The skin and the CNS, which both share a common ectodermal origin |

## NEUROFIBROMATOSIS

| | |
|---|---|
| **What is the mode of transmission of neurofibromatosis?** | Autosomal dominant transmission with high penetrance and variable expressivity, 50% are sporadic mutations. |
| **What is the prevalence?** | About 1 in 3,000 |
| **What is the eponym for neurofibromatosis?** | von Recklinghausen's disease |
| **What are the major differences between neurofibromatosis types 1 and 2?** | Type 1: predominantly peripheral lesions (e.g., cutaneous neurofibromas, cafe au lait spots)<br>Type 2: mostly intracranial manifestations, especially bilateral acoustic neuromas |
| **What is the most significant similarity between the two types?** | Both have increased risk of other CNS tumors |

| | |
|---|---|
| **What are two names for the peripheral nerve tumors of neurofibromatosis?** | Schwannoma and neurofibroma |
| **Are they histologically distinguishable?** | Usually, but their histological distinctions are not clinically important |
| **What is the common cellular element of schwannomas and neurofibromas?** | Both are composed of Schwann cells |
| **What is the distinction between them?** | Schwannomas are encapsulated. |
| **What are the classic skin, eye, and CNS findings of neurofibromatosis type 1?** | Skin—cafe au lait spots, neurofibromas<br>Eyes—Lisch nodules<br>CNS—schwannomas |
| **What is the significance of axillary freckles?** | They are seen in patients with neurofibromatosis type 1 |
| **What are Lisch nodules, what are their significance, and how frequently are they identified?** | Lisch nodules are symptomless pigmented hamartomas of the iris found in 100% of patients with neurofibromatosis by age 60. |
| **What is a common skeletal abnormality associated with neurofibromatosis type 1?** | Kyphoscolioses (however, pseudoarthrosis, scoliosis, and absence of the greater sphenoidal wing may also occur) |
| **What is the treatment for neurofibromatosis?** | Treatment is always symptomatic (e.g., shunting procedures, resection of symptomatic neurofibromas). |
| **What deformed the Elephant Man?** | A plexiform neurofibroma |

## TUBEROUS SCLEROSIS

| | |
|---|---|
| **What are three prominent clinical features of tuberous sclerosis?** | 1. Mental retardation<br>2. Seizure disorder<br>3. Adenoma sebaceum |

| | |
|---|---|
| **What is the mode of transmission?** | Autosomal dominant with variable penetrance and expressivity; also, it may occur as a new mutation. |
| **What is the prevalence?** | About 1 per 10,000 |
| **What are five major organs involved in tuberous sclerosis?** | 1. Brain<br>2. Skin<br>3. Retina<br>4. Kidneys<br>5. Heart |
| **What portion of the nervous system is not involved in tuberous sclerosis?** | Peripheral nervous system |
| **What are the four typical skin findings in tuberous sclerosis?** | 1. Adenoma sebaceum (facial angiofibromas)<br>2. Periungual fibromas<br>3. Shagreen patches (smooth plaques)<br>4. Hypopigmented patches (ash-leaf spots) |
| **What skin finding is most common?** | Ash-leaf spots |
| **What equipment may be needed to see ash-leaf spots?** | An ultraviolet Wood's lamp |
| **What skin finding is pathognomonic?** | Periungual or subungual fibromas, which are present in about 25% of patients |
| **What is the appearance of the typical eye finding?** | Mulberry phakomas, which are retinal hamartomas that project out of the retina on fundoscopic exam; they are present in about 50% of patients |
| **What is the most common presenting symptom in tuberous sclerosis?** | Seizures—in 80% to 90% of patients |
| **What are "tubers?"** | Cortical glial nodules that appear as smooth bumps on the cortical surface and also occur in subependymal regions |

**What is their appearance on CT and MRI?**

On CT, they appear as multiple areas of periventricular subependymal calcification. On MRI, they appear as multiple soft tissue tumors.

**What is the typical malignant CNS tumor in tuberous sclerosis?**

Subependymal giant cell astrocytomas may arise from subependymal tubers.

**What is the typical heart lesion?**

Benign rhabdomyoma

**What is its clinical significance?**

It is present in 50% of infants with tuberous sclerosis, and it causes about 25% of infant deaths in tuberous sclerosis due to obstruction of blood flow.

**What are typical kidney lesions?**

Angiomyolipomas and renal cysts

**What are their manifestations?**

Flank pain and hematuria

**What is the treatment for tuberous sclerosis?**

Symptomatic therapy
Anticonvulsants
Excision of tumors causing hydrocephalus

## VON HIPPEL-LINDAU DISEASE

**Why is it called a neuroectodermal disorder?**

It usually involves the cerebellum and retina.

**What is its cerebellar manifestation?**

Cerebellar hemangioblastoma

**What is its ophthalmic manifestation?**

Retinal hemangioblastoma or hemangioma

**Are there skin lesions?**

Rarely there are skin capillary nevi

**What are three characteristic pathologic findings in von Hippel-Lindau disease?**

Retinal and cerebellar **hemangioblastomas**
Pancreatic, renal, and epididymal **cysts**
Renal **carcinoma**

**What is the mode of inheritance?**

Autosomal dominant with high penetrance

**What are the pathologic criteria for von Hippel-Lindau disease?**

CNS or retinal hemangioblastoma and either one or more of the previous listed pathologic findings, or having a direct relative with the disease

**What is often the earliest *clinical* manifestation?**

Benign retinal hemangiomas

**What are the typical clinical manifestations of cerebellar hemangioblastomas?**

Symptoms are the same as for other posterior fossa tumors, mainly headache, nausea and vomiting, ataxia, dysarthria, and nystagmus.

**What are two possible vascular abnormalities of the retina?**

Hemangioma and hemangioblastoma

**Distinguish between hemangioma and hemangioblastoma.**

Hemangioma is a malformation, whereas hemangioblastoma is a neoplasm.

**What are two possible sites of hemangioblastoma in von Hippel-Lindau disease?**

Cerebellum and retina

**Which neuroimaging techniques are best for their identification?**

MRI or *contrasted* CT readily demonstrates these lesions.

**What renal lesions may be seen in von Hippel-Lindau disease?**

Simple or multilocular renal cysts, benign adenomas, hemangiomas, hypernephromas, or renal carcinomas

**How is the diagnosis established?**

Diagnosis is based on the clinical, radiographic, and pathologic findings as well as a positive family history.

**How is von Hippel-Lindau disease treated?**

Treatment is symptomatic.

## STURGE-WEBER SYNDROME

**What is the underlying pathologic abnormality in Sturge-Weber syndrome?**

Nonhereditary congenital malformation of the venous system of the head, eye, face, and CNS (leptomeningeal angiomatosis)

**What is the characteristic dermatologic manifestation?**

Port-wine stain—a facial nevus consisting of a venous angioma of the upper portion of the face that is usually on one side

**What is the characteristic ocular manifestation?**

Glaucoma, resulting in buphthalmos (i.e., enlargement of the eye)

**What is the characteristic CNS lesion?**

Angiomata of the leptomeninges of one hemisphere, usually ipsilateral to port-wine stain

**What is the most common neurologic manifestation?**

Seizures occur in up to 90% of patients. Patients also may have hemiparesis, hemianopsia, and mental retardation.

**What is the classic radiographic finding in Sturge-Weber syndrome?**

Railroad-track images of the underlying cerebral gyri seen on plain films

**What causes them?**

Calcification of the leptomeningeal angioma

**What treatment is available?**

Treatment of symptoms, especially for seizures, is the only therapy available.

**Is there neurologic significance to venous nevi of the second and third divisions of the trigeminal nerve?**

No

# 37

## Progressive Encephalopathy of Childhood

## BASIC CONSIDERATIONS

**What distinguishes a progressive encephalopathy from static encephalopathy?**

Static encephalopathy of any cause does not change over time; progressive encephalopathy is associated with neurologic deterioration.

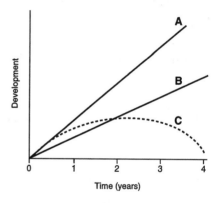

**Courses of childhood development**

A  Normal development
B  Static encephalopathy
C  Progressive neurodegenerative disease

**Characterize the developmental milestones in progressive encephalopathies of childhood.**

Early life: slow acquisition of developmental milestones
Later: regression of developmental milestones

**List four types of diseases that cause progressive encephalopathy of childhood.**

1. Leukodystrophies
2. Poliodystrophies (storage diseases)
3. Infectious diseases
4. Biochemical disorders

| | |
|---|---|
| **Are most of these syndromes acquired or inherited?** | Inherited |
| **What is the most common mode of inheritance?** | Autosomal recessive |
| **Divide these disorders into four groups based on primary anatomic location of pathology.** | 1. Those primarily affecting cortex<br>2. Those primarily affecting white matter<br>3. Those primarily affecting both white matter and cortex<br>4. Those primarily affecting basal ganglia |
| **What early manifestations characterize those disorders primarily affecting the cortex?** | Decline in *cognitive* development disproportionate to motor decline; seizures |
| **What early manifestations characterize those disorders primarily affecting the white matter?** | Decline in *motor* development disproportionate to cognitive decline; early spasticity |
| **What early manifestations characterize those primarily affecting the basal ganglia?** | Movement disorders, such as dystonia, tremor, and chorea |
| **What is another name for those disorders affecting primarily the white matter?** | Leukodystrophies |

## LEUKODYSTROPHIES

| | |
|---|---|
| **Name two types of leukodystrophies.** | 1. Metachromatic leukodystrophy (MLD)<br>2. Adrenal leukodystrophy (ALD) |
| **What other organ is affected in ALD?** | Adrenal gland |

## POLIODYSTROPHIES (STORAGE DISEASES)

| | |
|---|---|
| **What anatomic area is primarily affected by most storage diseases?** | Cortex (more so than white matter) |

| | |
|---|---|
| **Why do storage diseases result in storage of something?** | An inherited enzyme deficiency prevents the normal metabolic breakdown of the stored product (i.e., the stored product accumulates) |
| **What non-neurologic signs help in diagnosis of many storage diseases?** | Organomegaly or retinal changes caused by deposition of the storage product in cells in these areas |
| **How are storage diseases definitively diagnosed?** | Biochemical assay of blood sample demonstrates the enzyme deficiency or tissue biopsy demonstrates excess stored product |
| **Who usually gets Tay-Sachs disease, a gangliosidosis?** | People of Ashkenazi Jewish ancestry |
| **What is another name for Tay-Sachs disease?** | Gangliosidoses type II |
| **How is it definitively diagnosed?** | Biochemical assay for hexosaminidase A deficiency |
| **How is Gaucher's disease, a sphingolipidosis, definitively diagnosed?** | Biochemical assay for $\beta$-galactosidase deficiency |
| **What product is stored in Batten's disease?** | Lipofuscin—Batten's disease is one of the lipofuscinoses |
| **How is it definitively diagnosed?** | Demonstration of lipofuscin in tissue biopsy |
| **Name two progressive encephalopathies of childhood that cause megalocephaly.** | 1. Canavan's disease (cortex) 2. Alexander's disease (cortex and white matter) |

## INFECTIOUS DISEASES

| | |
|---|---|
| **Name one infectious, rapidly progressive encephalopathy of childhood.** | Subacute sclerosing panencephalitis (SSPE) |

| | |
|---|---|
| **What causes SSPE?** | Persistent infection by the measles virus; occurs very infrequently after immunization |
| **What class of disease is SSPE?** | Slow virus infection |
| **Who gets SSPE?** | Children 5 to 10 years of age |
| **Is SSPE common?** | No, not since widespread measles immunization |

## BIOCHEMICAL DISORDERS

| | |
|---|---|
| **Name three biochemical disorders other than storage diseases, which, if untreated, result in progressive encephalopathy.** | 1. Mitochondrial disorders<br>2. Amino acidurias<br>3. Organic acidurias |
| **What is a mitochondrion?** | Intracellular organelle involved in energy production |
| **What cells have mitochondria?** | All cells, except for mature erythrocytes |
| **What is mitochondrial inheritance?** | Inheritance passed via mitochondrial DNA |
| **In what ways is this different from chromosomal inheritance?** | 1. Exclusive use of cytoplasmic rather than nuclear (chromosomal) DNA<br>2. Inheritance is exclusively through the mother |
| **Is there always a family history of disease?** | No—cases may be sporadic |
| **What clinical features help distinguish mitochondrial diseases from other progressive encephalopathies of childhood?** | Intermittent or acute symptoms |

| | |
|---|---|
| **What is MELAS?** | A syndrome of **M**itochondrial **E**ncephalopathy, **L**actic **A**cidosis, and **S**troke |
| **What is MERRF?** | A syndrome of **M**itochondrial **E**ncephalopathy with **R**agged **R**ed **F**ibers |
| **What are ragged red fibers?** | Degenerating mitochondria seen histologically on biopsy (usually muscle) |
| **List four laboratory tests indicated in the workup of a possible mitochondrial disease.** | Lactate, pyruvate, alanine, urinary organic acids |
| **How are amino and organic acid metabolism defects diagnosed?** | Quantitative measurement of urine and serum amino and organic acids |
| **What amino aciduria is associated with stroke in infancy and childhood?** | Homocystinuria |
| **What classic amino aciduria presents in early life in blue-eyed, blond-haired children with a musty smell and static encephalopathy and is treated with dietary restrictions?** | Phenylketonuria (PKU) |

## PROGRESSIVE ENCEPHALOPATHIES PRIMARILY AFFECTING THE BASAL GANGLIA

| | |
|---|---|
| **Name three progressive childhood encephalopathies that primarily affect the basal ganglia.** | 1. Wilson's disease<br>2. Hallervorden-Spatz disease<br>3. Pelizaeus-Merzbacher disease |
| **What disease does a child with elevated liver enzymes, brown discoloration of the rim of the cornea (Kayser-Fleischer ring), and movement disorder probably have?** | Wilson's disease |

## DIAGNOSIS

**What is the comprehensive workup of progressive encephalopathy of childhood after history and physical examination?**

Serum and urine amino acids—to check for amino aciduria

Serum and urine organic acids—to check for organic aciduria

Serum lactate and pyruvate—to check for mitochondrial diseases

Specific biochemical assay—to check for enzyme defects

Formal ophthalmologic examination for retinal abnormalities and Kayser-Fleischer rings

EEG—to check for some storage diseases and SSPE

Tissue biopsy—to check for storage and mitochondrial diseases

Consider chromosome analysis to check for chromosome disorder

**Why is it important to accurately diagnose progressive encephalopathies, despite their generally poor prognosis?**

Some are treatable, such as Wilson's disease, PKU, and other amino acidurias. Most are inherited, and accurate genetic counseling requires knowing the diagnosis. Most parents want to know what to expect (i.e., prognosis).

# 38

# Hydrocephalus, Macrocephaly, and Microcephaly

## HEAD CIRCUMFERENCE

**What is the relationship between normal head and body growth in infancy?**

Head circumference should increase in proportion to body length.

**Following the *rules of 3s*, what is normal head circumference:**

  **At birth?**

35 cm

  **At 3 months of age?**

40 cm

  **At 9 months of age?**

45 cm

  **At 3 years of age?**

50 cm

  **As an adult?**

55 cm

**How can you remember this?**

By the "rule of 3s"—head circumference increases by 5 cm at each of the above noted intervals, which are multiples of 3

## MECHANISMS OF HYDROCEPHALUS

**Define hydrocephalus.**

Excessive intracranial CSF

**Where is the excessive CSF usually located?**

Intraventricular

**What is the consequence of hydrocephalus before cranial sutures fuse.**

Macrocephaly

**What is the consequence after cranial sutures fuse?**

Increased intracranial pressure (ICP)

| | |
|---|---|
| **What does disproportion indicate as a cause of poor development?** | Poor development is likely due to brain pathology. |
| **List three mechanisms of hydrocephalus. (Also see p. 312)** | 1. Excessive CSF production (rare)—e.g., from a choroid plexus papilloma<br>2. Obstruction of normal CSF pathways (90%)—e.g., from a congenital aqueductal stenosis or Arnold-Chiari malformation<br>3. Poor CSF absorption—e.g., from impaired arachnoid villi function as a complication of subarachnoid hemorrhage or meningitis |
| **Where is choroid plexus located?** | All four ventricles |
| **Where are arachnoid villi located?** | Scattered across the surface of the brain in the arachnoid (especially adjacent to venous channels) |
| **Trace the route of CSF from choroid plexus in lateral ventricle to arachnoid villi.** | Through interventricular foramen to third ventricle, through aqueduct to fourth ventricle, through foramina of Magendie and Luschka to subarachnoid space, and percolation across surfaces of brain to arachnoid villi |

## TYPES OF HYDROCEPHALUS

| | |
|---|---|
| **What is the mechanism of obstructive (or noncommunicating) hydrocephalus?** | Obstruction in CSF pathway within the ventricular system |
| **What is the classic clinical picture of an infant with congenital obstructive hydrocephalus?** | Large head, small face, and prominent forehead |
| **What is the mechanism of communicating hydrocephalus?** | Open CSF pathway; impaired arachnoid absorption |
| **What is hydrocephalus ex-vacuo?** | Large ventricles as a result of atrophic brain |

| | |
|---|---|
| **What is the sunset sign?** | Apparent downward displaced eyes secondary to protruding forehead in hydrocephalus |
| **What are two other causes of early life macrocephaly besides hydrocephalus?** | Chronic subdural hematoma and brain tumor |
| **What is the surgical treatment for hydrocephalus?** | Ventriculoperitoneal shunt |

## ARNOLD-CHIARI MALFORMATION

| | |
|---|---|
| **What is the Arnold-Chiari malformation, type I?** | Downward displacement of cerebellum and medulla through the foramen magnum |
| **What is the Arnold-Chiari malformation, type II?** | Type I plus lumbosacral meningomyelocele and hydrocephalus |
| **What is a meningomyelocele?** | Congenital outpouching of midline CNS, including meninges, cord, and roots |
| **Where is it most commonly located?** | Lumbosacral vertebrae |
| **What is usual functional consequence of meningomyelocele?** | Flaccid paraplegia, plus bowel and bladder incontinence |
| **Which is more common, Arnold-Chiari type I or II?** | Type II |
| **When does type I usually present as clinical hydrocephalus?** | Early adulthood |
| **Does it cause macrocephaly?** | No, because it becomes symptomatic after the skull fuses |
| **What does it cause?** | Increased ICP due to dilated ventricles |

## DANDY-WALKER SYNDROME

| | |
|---|---|
| **What is the Dandy-Walker malformation?** | Hydrocephalus with dilated fourth ventricle and large posterior fossa |

**What is the cause?**

Congenital malfunction of foramina of Luschka and Magendie

## MICROCEPHALY

**What is the usual cause of microcephaly?**

Small brain size due to brain pathology; or, rarely, it is inherited as a benign trait

**What is the relationship between brain and skull size?**

Brain size determines skull size.

# 39

# Attention Deficit Hyperactivity Disorder

**Define attention deficit disorder.**

Inability to attend to any task for an age-appropriate period of time

**Define hyperactivity.**

Inability to remain still for an appropriate period of time

**Do hyperactivity and attention deficit disorder coexist?**

Sometimes–this is known as attention deficit hyperactivity disorder (ADHD)

**When is it most likely to become apparent?**

Start of school years

**Which sex predominates?**

Males : Females = 3:1

**Is there a relationship between ADHD and intellect?**

No

**Is there a familial tendency?**

Yes—it is often inherited father to son

**When is pharmacotherapy indicated?**

When ADHD interferes with schooling, interpersonal relationships, or self-esteem

**What drugs may be helpful?**

Stimulants such as methylphenidate or amphetamines; clonidine, an alpha agonist

**Is there any risk associated with treatment with stimulants?**

Questionable risk of promoting subsequent development of tics or Tourette's syndrome

**Does methylphenidate put a child at risk for addiction?**

No, but there is risk of diversion to illicit uses

**What is the usual benefit?**

It aids concentration

**What is its most frequent side effect in a child?**

Appetite suppression and weight loss

**What are the physician's other important responsibilities to these children?**

Investigate other possible causes for poor performance:
Parental child-rearing skills
Environment
Intellect
Vision
Hearing

**What is the physician's most important responsibility to these children?**

Educate the child, parents, and teachers about ADD

# 40

# Autism and Pervasive Developmental Disorder

| | |
|---|---|
| **Name two conditions included among the pervasive developmental disorders.** | Autism<br>Asperger's disorder |
| **What type of disorder are they?** | Behavioral disorder |
| **At what age do they first present?** | Before age 3 years |
| **Are there biologic or radiologic markers?** | No |
| **Characterize the diagnostic behavior.** | Inadequate social interactions |
| **Give some childhood examples.** | Failure to respond, point, show, play with others; poor eye contact, smile; disinterest in affection |
| **Characterize verbal and non-verbal communication.** | Sparse |
| **Characterize adaptability.** | Poor. Prefer routine |
| **How is autism diagnosed?** | Neuropsychological screen |
| **List four differential diagnoses.** | Mental retardation, deafness, tuberous sclerosis, lead encephalopathy |
| **How is it treated?** | Multifactorial education |
| **Does treatment make a difference?** | Yes |

**What is an autistic savant?**
Autism with unusual specific ability, such as calculation

**What is an outdated term for this ability?**
"Idiot savant," a poor term because autism does not equal low IQ

# 41

# Child Abuse: Non-Accidental Trauma

**What child abuse injury is most associated with death or serious long-term sequelae?**

Subdural hematoma (SDH), 80% of which are bilateral in child abuse cases

**What is the mechanism of injury in child abuse-related SDH?**

Acceleration–deceleration injury (i.e., shaking)

**What is the vernacular term?**

Shaken baby

**When do you suspect a shaken baby?**

Lethargic child with multiple bruises or fractures of varying age, with or without seizures

**What symptoms indicate the shaken baby has an SDH?**

Lethargy progressing to coma and evidence of increased ICP

**What are three key neurologic physical findings associated with shaken baby syndrome?**

1. Retinal hemorrhages
2. Large head circumference
3. Bulging fontanelle

**What three characteristics of plain skull radiographs suggest child abuse rather than other trauma?**

1. Multiple fractures
2. Bilateral fractures
3. Fractures across sutures

**What are some of the long-term sequelae of repeated CNS injury caused by child abuse?**

Mental retardation, seizures, hydrocephalus, ataxia

**What is the single most important preventative intervention in suspected child abuse?**

Notify Social Services, so that the child is protected from further injury

# Section VI

Diagnostic Procedures in Neurology

# 42

# Basis of Neuroimaging

## MRI

| | |
|---|---|
| **What does MRI stand for?** | Magnetic resonance imaging |
| **Does MRI use x-rays?** | No |
| **List three advantages of MRI over CT for neuroimaging.** | 1. Minimal distortion by bone<br>2. Clearer visualization of the anatomy<br>3. Ability to obtain images through any plane |
| **What are the three most common planes (or "cuts") obtained by MRI?** | 1. Sagittal<br>2. Coronal<br>3. Horizontal (also called axial, or transverse) [see figure on p. 306] |
| **What conditions may prevent a successful MRI?** | Severe claustrophobia<br>Ferromagnetic object in brain, eye, or heart<br>Inability to lie still<br>Cardiac pacemaker |
| **What strategies minimize some of these restrictions?** | Sedation; use of an open imaging machine |
| **How does MRI work?** | Tissue hydrogen protons are oriented and then subjected to radiofrequency waves in a magnetic field. Their energy radiation is read to create the images. |
| **Where are most hydrogen protons?** | Water |
| **What does the _T_ in a T1 image represent?** | The time necessary for a tissue's protons to orient parallel to a magnetic pulse |

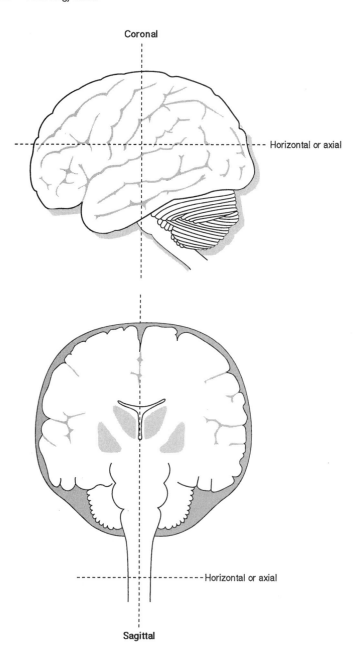

| | |
|---|---|
| **What does the _T_ in a T2 image represent?** | The time necessary for tissue to decay from full magnetization |
| **Name the five most useful settings in MRI of the brain and spinal cord.** | 1. Tl<br>2. T2<br>3. Proton density<br>4. FLAIR (**F**luid **A**ttenuated **I**nversion **R**ecovery)<br>5. DWI (diffusion weighted) |
| **What color is CSF on Tl images?** | Black |
| **What color is CSF on T2 settings?** | White |
| **What color is air on either setting?** | Black |
| **What color is cortical bone (skull)?** | It is not visualized. |
| **Why?** | Most protons are in water, and bone has no water. |
| **What three factors determine the appearance of blood on an MRI?** | 1. Imaging sequence (T1, T2, etc)<br>2. Whether the blood is flowing<br>3. The age of a clot |
| **What color is blood flowing in vessels?** | Black |
| **Name four stages of a hematoma as distinguished by MRI.** | 1. Hyperacute (< 24 hours)<br>2. Acute (1–3 days)<br>3. Subacute (3 days–3 weeks)<br>4. Chronic (> 3 weeks) |
| **Why must DWI be compared to beta zero or T2 images?** | To detect a normal "shine through" signal that can appear as a pathological DWI signal |
| **What is best visualized by each sequence below:**<br>**T1?**<br>**T2?**<br>**FLAIR?**<br>**DWI?** | <br><br>Normal brain parenchymal structures<br>Edema, infarct, tumor, demyelination<br>Gliosis, edema, infarct<br>Acute infarct |

| | |
|---|---|
| **What two conditions appear as T2 multifocal subcortical white spots?** | MS plaques and multifocal ischemia |
| **Name the contrast agents used in MRI.** | Gadolinium compounds |
| **What does gadolinium enhancement indicate?** | Breakdown of blood–brain barrier |
| **Can an MRI be used during pregnancy?** | There are insufficient data to permit routine use at present, although it is thought to be safe and can be used in emergencies. |
| **What is MRA?** | Magnetic resonance angiography, which is similar to MRI, but the acquisition sequences and image reconstruction are designed to visualize blood vessels |

## COMPUTERIZED TOMOGRAPHY (CT)

| | |
|---|---|
| **What is "computed tomography"?** | Tomography is the process of obtaining radiographic images in a cross-sectional plane through an object (similar to slicing through an orange). The brain or spinal cord is surveyed by a series of narrow radiograph beams originating in a 360° circle around the patient. A computer then reconstructs these images. |
| **How is a head CT performed?** | The patient is placed in a gantry that circumnavigates the head and obtains radiographs of the brain. It neither hurts nor does it require manipulation of the patient, unless contrast is used. |
| **How is this method of obtaining images fundamentally different from MRI?** | MRI uses a magnetic field and radiofrequency waves, whereas CT uses x-rays. |
| **What color is normal brain substance on CT?** | Various shades of grey |

**Why are some substances white on CT?**

They are radiopaque. The terms *radiopaque* and *hyperdense* are used interchangeably. Both terms are analogous to increased signal intensity (white) in MRI.

**What three substances are hyperdense on brain CT?**

1. Calcium
2. Standing blood
3. Metal

**Name a normal and a pathologic circumstance in which calcium would be seen on brain CT.**

Calcium is normally present in bone, and it may be present in tumors.

**Name a pathologic circumstance in which blood would be seen on CT.**

Extravascular blood (e.g., in intracerebral hematoma or subarachnoid hemorrhage)

**Name a normal and a pathologic circumstance in which metal would be seen on brain CT.**

Metal may "normally" be present in dental fillings, and may pathologically be present in aneurysm clips or foreign bodies.

**Is CT or MRI better for assessing suspected acute intracranial bleeding?**

CT

**Why?**

Acute blood, especially subarachnoid hemorrhage, is usually easier to see on CT.

**What is contrast?**

An iodinated radiopaque substance injected intravenously before obtaining CT images.

**What is contrast enhancement?**

Increased density (enhancement) in a region of blood–brain barrier breakdown

**What three conditions typically demonstrate contrast enhancement?**

Tumor, abscess, and sometimes subacute cerebral infarcts

**What are the potential complications of CT?**

Radiation exposure; however, the amount of exposure is much less than a routine chest radiograph

**What are contraindications to CT?**

Pregnancy is a contraindication, because even small doses of radiation are potentially harmful to a fetus. When CT is necessary during pregnancy, the abdomen can be shielded to reduce exposure of the fetus.

## CEREBRAL ANGIOGRAPHY

**What is a cerebral angiogram (cerebral arteriogram)?**
Radiographs of cerebral vessels after injection of a radiopaque contrast material

**How is a cerebral angiogram performed?**
The usual approach is through the femoral artery; a catheter is threaded over a guide wire, up the aorta, and into the carotid or vertebral arteries. Contrast material, usually a water-based iodine compound, is injected through the catheter. Sequential radiograph images are obtained in different planes and after different time intervals for arterial and venous images.

**What are the risks of cerebral angiography?**
Local bleeding or hematoma
Infection
Arterial lacerations
Pseudoaneurysm formation
Renal failure
Stroke or TIA
Contrast reactions (e.g., allergic reaction, contrast encephalopathy)
Rarely, death

**What is the risk of stroke?**
Less than 1%

**What are four vascular abnormalities best diagnosed by cerebral angiogram?**
1. Aneurysms
2. Arteriovenous malformations
3. Cerebral sinus thrombosis
4. Arterial stenosis

**What are five causes of arterial luminal stenosis or occlusion identifiable by cerebral angiography?**
1. Atherosclerosis
2. Thrombosis
3. Embolism
4. Dissection
5. Vasculitis

**What are some therapeutic uses for angiography?**

Embolization of aneurysms, intra-arterial/intracranial thrombolysis, large vessel angioplasty, embolization of blood supply to tumors or arteriovenous malformations (AVMs)

**What other diagnostic studies can sometimes be used in the place of cerebral angiography?**

MRI for AVMs, tumors, sinus thrombosis and vessel dissections
MRA for vessel anatomy and dissection
Head CT with contrast for tumors and their vascular supply

**In whom is cerebral angiography relatively contraindicated?**

Any patient with severe contrast allergies

**What prophylactic medication reduces risk of contrast reaction?**

Steroids

**What advantage does MRA have over conventional angiography?**

It is less invasive and free of risk.

**What is a limitation of MRA?**

It is not able to visualize small vessels.

**What vascular pathology is better visualized by MRA?**

Carotid dissection

## MYELOGRAPHY (INCLUDING CT MYELOGRAPHY)

**What is myelography?**

Plain radiographic and fluoroscopic visualization of the silhouettes of spinal cord and nerve roots by radiopaque contrast media injected into the subarachnoid space

**What is CT myelography?**

Transverse CT imaging of spinal cord and nerve roots after contrast injection

**How is CT myelography performed?**

Water soluble iodine-based contrast material is injected by lumbar puncture into the subarachnoid space. Plain radiography and CT scan then visualizes the silhouette of the spinal cord and the nerve roots; CT allows for some visualization of the soft tissues surrounding or impinging on these structures.

**What are the risks involved in myelography?**

Bacterial meningitis
Chemical arachnoiditis
Seizures
Headaches
Nausea
Vomiting
Bleeding or infection

**What are the indications for CT myelography?**

Suspected spinal cord or nerve root compression by herniated disc, osteophyte, or other mass; also, can indirectly show evidence of intramedullary lesion (i.e., spinal cord swelling) or localize level of subarachnoid block

**What test has superseded CT myelography, and why?**

MRI—it is safer, provides more information, and has fewer side effects and risks; it provides images of the intramedullary and extramedullary region of the spinal cord, and it visualizes soft and bony tissue around the spinal cord and nerve roots

**What are three limitations of CT myelography?**

1. It does not visualize the intramedullary aspects of the spinal cord well.
2. It requires lumbar puncture.
3. There is some risk of chemical arachnoiditis.

## CISTERNOGRAPHY AND VENTRICULOGRAPHY
(See also Chapter 38)

**What is radionuclide cisternography?**

Visualization of the CSF system performed by infusing a radionuclide marker into the CSF

**What is the normal pattern of CSF flow in and around the brain?**

Lateral ventricle to third ventricle, to cerebral aqueduct, to fourth ventricle, to basal cisterns, through incisura, across cerebral hemispheres, to arachnoid granulations

**How much CSF does the average brain contain?**

About 150 mL, of which 50 mL is in the ventricles; CSF is produced at a rate of 500 mL/day

**What are the clinical indications for cisternography?**

Evaluation of hydrocephalus (communicating versus noncommunicating), especially normal pressure hydrocephalus (NPH)

**What is the difference between communicating and noncommunicating hydrocephalus?**

In communicating hydrocephalus, there is no mechanical obstruction in the ventricular or subarachnoid system, whereas in noncommunicating hydrocephalus there is. Communicating hydrocephalus usually occurs because there is decreased absorption by the arachnoid granulations (rarely increased production by the ependyma).

**Is NPH communicating or noncommunicating?**

Communicating

**What is the typical result of radionuclide cisternography in NPH?**

Early entry of radiotracer into the ventricles with persistence after 24–48 hrs (long) and with delayed movement across the cerebral hemispheres

**What test has superseded radionuclide ventriculography/ cisternography?**

MRI—however, it is an anatomic test and does not demonstrate the physiologic properties of the CSF

**What is the typical MRI picture of NPH?**

Ventriculomegaly with transependymal diffusion of CSF

## SINGLE PHOTON EMISSION COMPUTERIZED TOMOGRAPHY (SPECT)

**What does SPECT measure?**

Regional cerebral blood flow

**How is SPECT performed?**

A radioactive substance is injected intravenously, and the pattern of radiation is detected and reconstructed by CT.

**What is SPECT used for?**    To help localize site of seizure onset

**What finding on interictal SPECT localizes a seizure focus?**    Focal decreased uptake signaling hypoperfusion

**What finding on ictal SPECT localizes a seizure focus?**    Focal increased uptake signaling hyperperfusion

**What complicates the use of ictal SPECT?**    Radionuclide must be injected within 90 seconds of seizure onset.

**Why is quick administration important?**    Once the seizure spreads, the findings become less focal.

## POSITRON EMISSION TOMOGRAPHY (PET)

**What does PET, using 18-F-2 deoxyglucose (FDG), measure?**    Regional cerebral glucose metabolism

**How is PET performed?**    Radioisotope is linked to a molecule, which is injected intravenously.

**For what is PET indicated?**    1. To help localize site of seizure onset
2. To distinguish between neoplasm and postradiation necrosis

**What PET finding distinguishes malignancy from radiation necrosis?**    Malignancy—hypermetabolism due to increased cellular activity
Postradiation necrosis—hypometabolism due to decreased cellular activity

**Although PET is a more specific and sensitive functional test than SPECT, what limits more widespread use of PET?**    A cyclotron is needed to generate short half-life isotopes for PET.

## NONINVASIVE CAROTID EVALUATION (NICE)

**What is another name for NICE studies?**    Carotid Doppler examination

**What signal does NICE use?**

Ultrasonic Doppler

**What does it measure?**

Blood flow velocity; the vessel wall may also be directly visualized for abnormalities

**When is it an appropriate test in evaluation of stroke?**

To screen for suspected carotid stenosis or anterior circulation thromboembolus

**What NICE finding corresponds with significant stenosis?**

High flow velocity

**What is the finding in total occlusion?**

No measurable flow
NICE cannot distinguish between no-flow (occlusion) and extremely low-flow (tight stenosis with patent vessel) conditions; angiography is necessary

# 43

## Looking at Neuroimages

**Note:** This chapter is divided into 11 exercises, each of which is based on a neuroimage.

**What are the three most common planes (or "cuts") obtained by MRI?**

1. Sagittal
2. Coronal
3. Axial (also called horizontal or transverse) (see p. 306)

**What is the standard right–left orientation of all neuroradiologic images?**

The right side of the object is on the left side of the picture.

### EXERCISE I

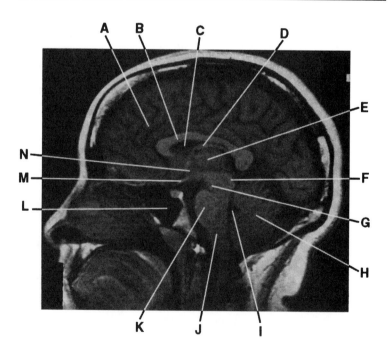

**What type of neuroimaging study is this?**

Sagittal head MRI

**Is this T1- or T2-weighted?**

T1

**How can you tell?**

In T1, CSF is black
In T2, CSF is white

**Is it contrast enhanced?**

No

**How can you tell?**

Intravenous gadolinium turns blood vessels white on T1 MRI (because of enhanced signal). They are black in this image. (Contrast is not useful in T2 images, because CSF is already white, so contrast cannot be seen.)

**For each letter on the image, name the anatomic structure it represents.**

A—cerebral cortex
B—corpus callosum
C—third ventricle
D—fornix
E—thalamus
F—midbrain tectum
G—midbrain tegmentum
H—cerebellum
I—fourth ventricle
J—medulla
K—pons
L—paranasal sinus
M—region of optic chiasm and tract
N—hypothalamus

## EXERCISE 2

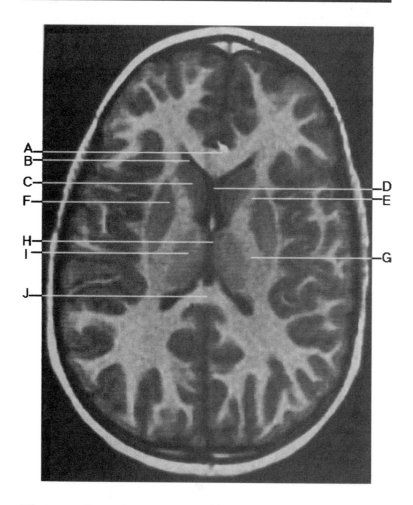

| | |
|---|---|
| **What type of neuroimaging study is this?** | Axial (or transverse) head MRI |
| **Is this T1- or T2-weighted?** | T1-weighted |
| **Is it contrast enhanced?** | No |
| **For each letter on the image, name the anatomic structure it represents.** | A—genu of corpus callosum<br>B—lateral ventricle<br>C—head of caudate nucleus<br>D—septum pellucidum |

E—anterior limb of internal capsule
F—globus pallidus and putamen
  (basal ganglia)
G—posterior limb of internal capsule
H—third ventricle
I—thalamus
J—splenium of corpus callosum

## EXERCISE 3

Image 3A

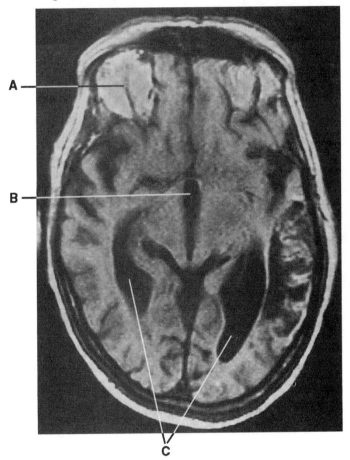

A

B

C

Image 3B

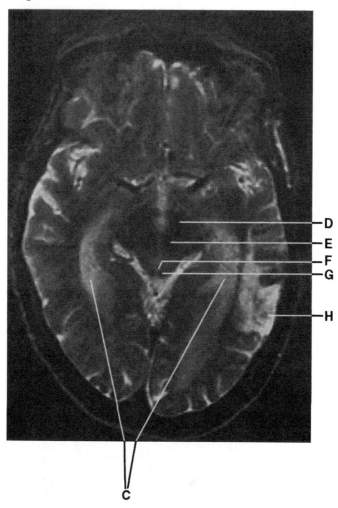

| | |
|---|---|
| **What type of neuroimaging studies are these?** | Axial head MRIs |
| **Is *image A* T1- or T2-weighted?** | *Image A* is T1-weighted. CSF is black. |
| **Is *image B* T1- or T2-weighted?** | *Image B* is T2-weighted. CSF is white. |

| | |
|---|---|
| **Are they contrast enhanced?** | No |
| **Why is one orbit larger than the other in *image A*?** | Because the patient's head is imperfectly positioned |
| **For each letter on the images, name the anatomic structure it represents.** | A—orbital contents<br>B—third ventricle<br>C—lateral ventricles<br>D—corticospinal tracts<br>E—red nucleus<br>F—cerebral aqueduct<br>G—midbrain tectum (corpora quadrigemina)<br>H—left parietal lobe |
| **Where is the pathology located?** | H—left parietal lobe |
| **What is the difference between the signal in the pathologic area on the T1 versus the T2 image?** | Decreased signal on T1 and increased signal on T2 |
| **What is the physiologic correlate of decreased T1 and increased T2 signal?** | Increased water, which may represent CSF, edema, proteinaceous cyst contents, or inflammation |
| **Which is most likely in this case?** | Proteinaceous material |
| **Is there any surrounding edema present?** | No |
| **Why is the adjacent ventricle enlarged (C)?** | Loss of brain parenchyma |
| **Is this lesion acute or chronic, and why?** | It is chronic because there is no surrounding edema to suggest an acute insult, and loss of brain parenchyma occurs over a long duration. |
| **What is the most likely diagnosis, and why?** | Chronic ischemic infarct (old stroke), because of focal cystic encephalomalacia in the area of brain supplied by a single vessel (the MCA in this case) |

## EXERCISE 4

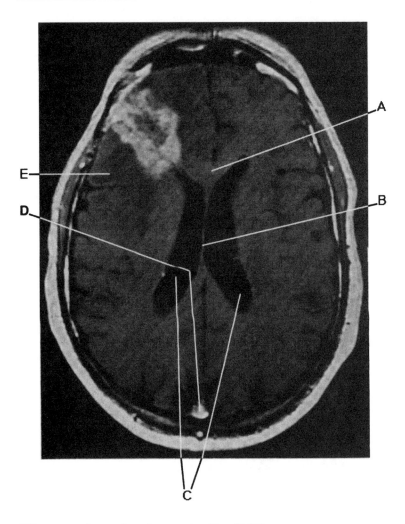

| | |
|---|---|
| **What type of neuroimaging study is this?** | Axial head MRI |
| **Is this T1- or T2-weighted?** | T1-weighted |
| **Is it contrast enhanced?** | Yes. There is contrast in the superior sagittal sinus (seen as increased signal in the posterior interhemispheric fissure; letter *D* in the image). |

| | |
|---|---|
| **For *letters A–E* on the image, name the anatomic structures represented.** | A—corpus callosum<br>B—septum pellucidum<br>C—lateral ventricles<br>D—sagittal sinus in cross-section<br>E—right frontal lobe |
| **Where is the pathology located?** | Right frontal lobe |
| **Describe the pattern of enhancement (increased signal).** | Enhancement is non-homogeneous, with the periphery enhancing more than the center ("ring enhancing") |
| **What does the surrounding area of decreased signal represent?** | Edema (*letter E* in image) |
| **Why does the margin of the lesion enhance?** | Breakdown of the blood–brain barrier |
| **What does the central area of decreased signal represent?** | Liquefying necrotic material |
| **What is the differential diagnosis of this lesion?** | Primary brain tumor, metastatic brain tumor, abscess |
| **What is a helpful distinguishing radiologic feature of metastatic brain tumor?** | Multiple lesions |
| **Can brain tumor be reliably distinguished from abscess radiologically?** | Not usually |
| **If this is primary brain tumor, what is the most likely pathologic diagnosis?** | Glioblastoma multiforme |

## EXERCISE 5

Image 5A

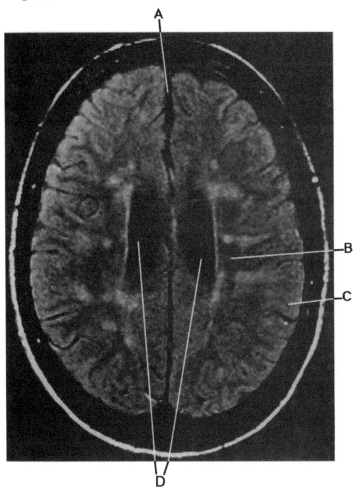

Image 5B

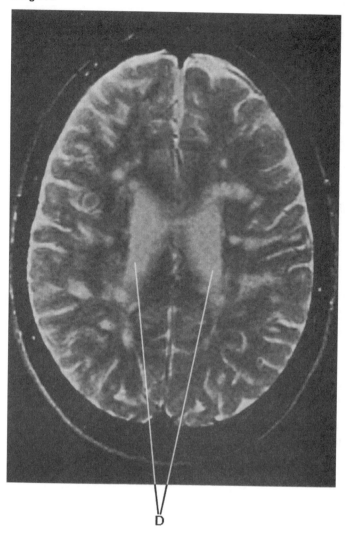

| | |
|---|---|
| **What type of neuroimaging studies are these?** | Axial head MRIs |
| **Is *image 5A* either T1- or T2-weighted?** | 5A is proton density; this best separates periventricular hyperintensities from CSF. |
| **Is *image B* T1- or T2-weighted?** | *Image B* is T2-weighted. |

**Are they enhanced?**

No

**For each letter on the images, name the anatomic structures it represents.**

A—interhemispheric fissure
B—white matter of corona radiata
C—cerebral cortex
D—lateral ventricle

**Where is the pathology located?**

White matter, primarily around the ventricles (i.e., periventricular)

**Describe the abnormal signal characteristics.**

Patchy increased signal on both images

**What white matter pathology is the most likely cause of this signal?**

Demyelination

**What is the etiologic differential diagnosis?**

MS; multiple small vessel strokes

**What is the most likely diagnosis, and why?**

MS—because the increased signal is primarily periventricular with finger-like extensions into the white matter perpendicular to the ventricle (Dawson's fingers)

**Can this be clearly differentiated from multiple infarcts entirely on the basis of its radiologic appearance?**

No. The diagnosis must be made using other factors, especially age.

## EXERCISE 6

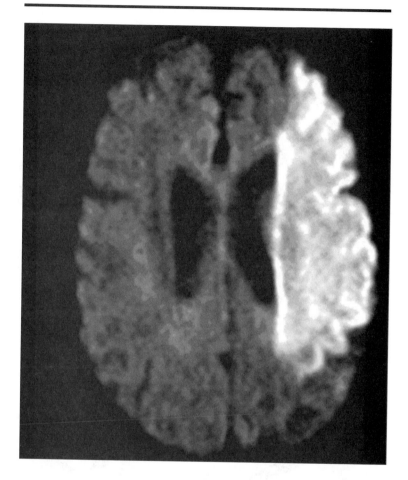

| | |
|---|---|
| **What type of neuroimaging study is this?** | Diffusion-weighted MRI |
| **Where is the abnormality?** | Left hemisphere |
| **What is the most likely pathology?** | Acute ischemic infarction |
| **What arterial distribution is involved?** | Left middle cerebral artery |
| **What advantage does this have over other MRI sequences?** | Much earlier detection of acute infarction |

## EXERCISE 7

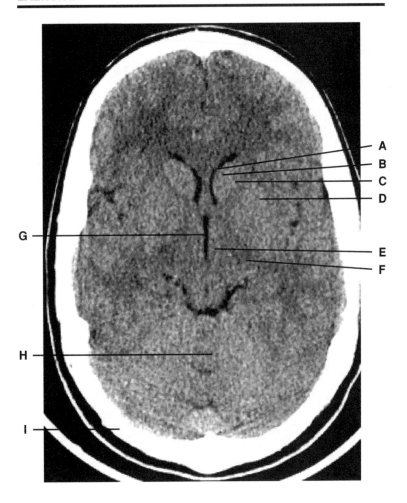

**What type of neuroimaging study is this?**

Axial CT (not MRI)

**Is this contrasted?**

No

**How can you tell?**

Intravenous iodinated contrast media causes hyperdensity (white) in blood vessels. Blood vessels in this image cannot be seen, because they are not filled with contrast.

**For each letter on the image, name the anatomic structure it represents.**

A—lateral ventricles
B—caudate nucleus
C—anterior limb of internal capsule
D—globus pallidus and putamen
   (lentiform nucleus)
E—thalamus
F—posterior limb of internal capsule
G—third ventricle
H—vermis of cerebellum
I—skull

**Which study gives better images of brain structure and pathology?**

MRI, except often for subarachnoid blood

## EXERCISE 8

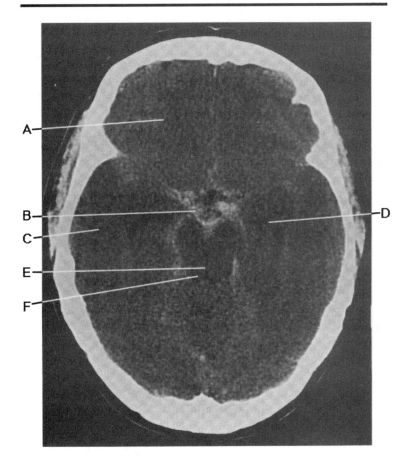

| | |
|---|---|
| **What type of neuroimaging study is this?** | Axial CT (not MRI) |
| **Is this contrasted?** | No |
| **For each letter on the image, name the anatomic structure it represents.** | A—frontal lobe cortex in anterior cranial fossa<br>B—suprasellar cistern<br>C—temporal lobe cortex in middle cranial fossa<br>D—dilated temporal horns of lateral ventricles<br>E—cerebral aqueduct<br>F—midbrain |
| **Where is the pathology located?** | Subarachnoid space, especially visible in the suprasellar cistern and outlining the brainstem (*letter B* in image) |
| **Describe the abnormal density characteristics of the suprasellar cistern.** | Hyperdense (B) |
| **What is the most likely pathophysiologic correlate of increased density in this case?** | Blood in the CSF |
| **What is the most likely radiologic diagnosis?** | Subarachnoid hemorrhage (SAH) |
| **What is the most likely etiology?** | Rupture of aneurysm |

## EXERCISE 9

**Note:** There are a total of three radiologic lesions with similar imaging characteristics in the following two images.

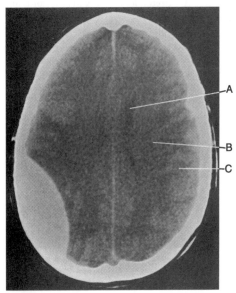

Image A

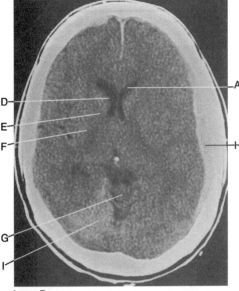

Image B

| | |
|---|---|
| **What type of neuroimaging studies are these?** | Axial CTs from two different patients |
| **Are they contrasted?** | No |
| **For *letters A–G* on these two images, name the anatomic structures represented.** | A—lateral ventricle<br>B—white matter of corona radiata<br>C—cerebral cortex<br>D—caudate nucleus<br>E—internal capsule<br>F—globus pallidus and putamen<br>G—vermis of cerebellum |
| **Where is the pathology located in *image A*?** | Right posterior region |
| **Where are the two sites of pathology in *image B*?** | Left parietal region and right cerebellum |
| **Describe the shape of the left parietal lesion in *image B*.** | Curved, following the inner surface of the skull (*letter H*) |
| **Describe the difference in shape between the pathology in *image A* and the parietal pathology in *image B*.** | *Image A*—convex or bulging into the brain<br>*Image B*—concave or lens-shaped (following the contour of the brain) |
| **Do the lesions in *images A* and *B* have an increased or decreased density?** | Increased |
| **What is the differential diagnosis of increased density on CT?** | Acute blood, calcium |
| **What does the increased density represent in these cases?** | Blood—it is not as bright as calcium and is an acute lesion with mass effect (effacement of the lateral ventricle and displacement of the underlying cortex) |
| **What are the most likely diagnoses of *images A* and *B*?** | *Image A*—epidural hematoma<br>*Image B*—subdural hematoma |
| **What is letter I in *image B*?** | SAH or tentorial subdural hematoma |
| **Describe its shape.** | Fan-shaped, in this instance |

## EXERCISE 10

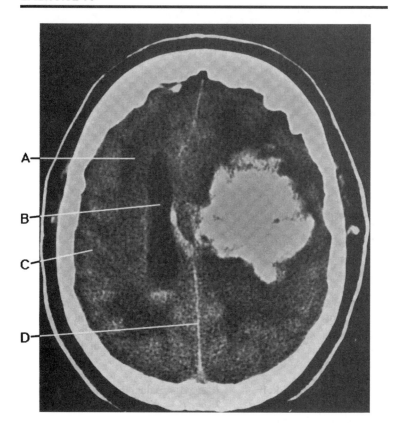

| | |
|---|---|
| **What type of neuroimaging study is this?** | Axial noncontrasted CT |
| **For each letter on the image, name the anatomic structure it represents.** | A—white matter of corona radiata<br>B—lateral ventricle<br>C—cerebral cortex<br>D—falx cerebri in the interhemispheric fissure |
| **Where is the most obvious pathology located?** | Left hemisphere |
| **Describe the density of the abnormality.** | Increased signal |
| **What is the most likely pathophysiologic correlate of increased density in this case?** | Blood |
| **What is the most likely radiologic diagnosis?** | Acute intracerebral hemorrhage (ICH) with mass effect, obliterating the left lateral ventricle and displacing it to the right. Hypodensity of the surrounding white matter represents edema, suggesting an acute lesion. |
| **What are the two most common causes of ICH?** | 1. Amyloid angiopathy<br>2. Hypertension |

## EXERCISE II

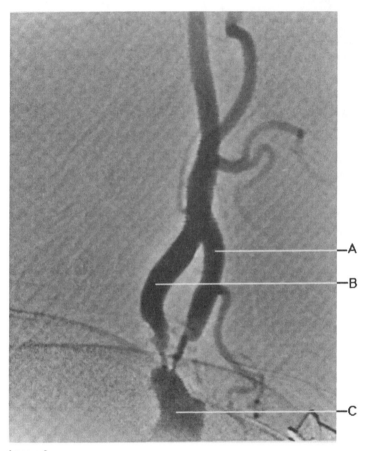

Image A

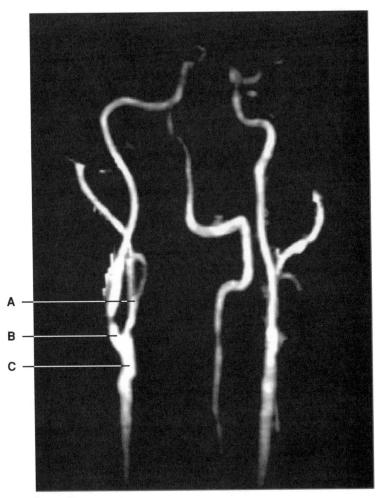

**Image B**

| | |
|---|---|
| **What type of neuroimaging study is *image A*?** | Carotid angiogram |
| **What type of neuroimaging study is *image B*?** | Magnetic resonance angiogram (MRA) |
| **In the images, what arteries do A, B, and C represent?** | A—external carotid artery<br>B—internal carotid artery<br>C—common carotid artery |

**How can you identify *letter A* as the external carotid artery?**

It branches in the neck shortly after arising from the common carotid bifurcation.

**Where is the pathology located in *image A*?**

Origin of both the external and internal carotid arteries, at the bifurcation of the common carotid artery

**Where is the pathology located in *image B*?**

It is located in the right internal carotid artery, near the bifurcation of the common carotid artery. The right vertebral artery is absent.

**Describe the abnormalities.**

Eccentric narrowing of the vessel lumens

**What is the most likely etiology?**

Atherosclerotic plaque

# 44 ___ Lumbar Puncture and CSF Analysis

| | |
|---|---|
| **At what vertebral level does the spinal cord end in adults?** | T12–L1 |
| **What spinal interspace is located at the level of the iliac crests in adults?** | L3–L4 or L4–L5 |
| **How is LP performed?** | Patient lies in lateral decubitus position and a needle is inserted between the spinous processes into the L3–L4 intervertebral space |
| **What is the upper normal limit for CSF opening pressure?** | 200 mm |
| **WBCs?** | 0–5 WBCs |
| **RBCs?** | 0–1,000 RBCs |
| **Protein?** | <60 mg/dl protein |
| **Glucose?** | ~80% of serum glucose, or 80 mg/dl |
| **When is LP indicated?** | When meningitis, subarachnoid hemorrhage, or pseudotumor cerebri is suspected |
| **What is the typical CSF profile in bacterial versus viral meningitis?** | See Chapter 22 |

Table 44–1.  CSF Findings in Bacterial and Viral Meningitis

| CSF Findings | Bacterial Meningitis | Viral Meningitis |
|---|---|---|
| Protein | Increased | Normal to increased |
| Glucose | Decreased | Normal |
| WBCs | Polymorphonuclear lymphocytes | Mononuclear lymphocytes |

**What two tests can lead to quick diagnosis of cryptococcal meningitis?**

India ink and cryptococcal antigen

**What are five contraindications to lumbar puncture (LP)?**

1. Thrombocytopenia
2. Infection at level of puncture
3. Papilledema
4. Cerebral mass lesion
5. Recent head trauma

**What is the most effective prevention of post-LP headache?**

Use of a small-bore spinal needle (20–22 gauge) (see Chapter 30)

**How long must blood be present in CSF before xanthochromia develops?**

2–4 hours

**What common endocrine abnormality often causes high CSF protein?**

Diabetes mellitus

**What is Froin's syndrome?**

High lumbar CSF protein below a block

**What confirming CSF test result helps diagnose probable MS?**

Oligoclonal bands present in CSF that are not present in serum

**Why?**

It indicates intrathecal production of antibodies, as occurs in MS

**What CSF test is a nonspecific marker of demyelination of any cause?**

Myelin basic protein

**What CSF test is a nonspecific and indirect indication of CNS inflammation?**

R value (ratio of total protein/albumin)

# 45

# Electromyography and Nerve Conduction Studies

**What does EMG stand for?**  Electromyography—it is also called "the needle exam"

**What does NCS stand for?**  Nerve conduction studies

**What is an EMG/NCS?**  An electrical assessment of muscle and nerve

**What types of disorders are assessed by EMG/NCS?**  Diseases of peripheral nerve, neuromuscular junction, and muscle

## EMG

**How is the electrical activity displayed in an EMG?**  The activity is displayed as waveforms on a display screen and as sound through a loudspeaker.

**How is the EMG performed?**  The physician places a needle electrode into selected muscles to evaluate the electrical activity produced during needle insertion, at rest, and with voluntary activation.

**What is the normal electrical activity seen in a resting muscle?**  None

**What abnormal activity may be seen in a denervated muscle at rest?**  Fasciculation potentials, fibrillation potentials, and positive sharp waves may arise spontaneously or following insertion of the needle electrode.

**Differentiate between fasciculation and fibrillation potentials.**  A fasciculation is the spontaneous depolarization of many muscle fibers belonging to a single motor unit and may be seen as visible muscle twitch, a fibrillation is the spontaneous depolarization of a *single* muscle fiber and cannot be seen clinically.

**What is meant by the term *motor unit*?**

A motor unit consists of an anterior horn cell, its axon, and the neuromuscular junctions and muscle fibers that it innervates.

**Name the electrical activity that arises from contracting muscle.**

Motor unit potentials (MUPs)

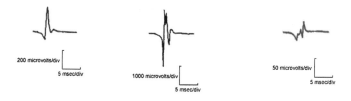

Normal MUP          Neuropathic MUP          Myopathic MUP

**What features of MUPs are routinely described?**

The size (amplitude and duration) and morphology (number of phases) of the waveforms

**How do MUPs appear in a neuropathic lesion, and why?**

MUPs are large and polyphasic. Damage to a motor axon denervates its muscles and abolishes its MUP. Adjacent undamaged motor axons sprout new terminals and reinnervate the denervated muscle fibers. This new motor unit now contains more muscle fibers and, therefore, produces a larger MUP.

**How do MUPs appear in a myopathic lesion, and why?**

MUPs are small and polyphasic. These result from the loss of muscle fibers and asynchronous firing of the remaining muscle fibers within each motor unit.

## NCS

**How are NCS performed?**

The physician or technician delivers a supramaximal electrical stimulus over a peripheral nerve to cause depolarization of the nerve fibers. The action potentials generated are evaluated.

**How does the technique differ for motor and sensory NCS?**

For motor NCS, the electrical stimulator is placed over a motor or mixed nerve, and the recording electrodes are placed over a distal muscle supplied by that nerve. For sensory NCS, the electrical stimulator is placed over a sensory or mixed nerve, and the recording electrodes are placed at a different site along the nerve.

**What is the term for the response recorded over a muscle?**

The compound muscle action potential (CMAP) is recorded over a muscle.

**Over a sensory nerve?**

The sensory nerve action potential (SNAP) is recorded over a nerve.

**Differentiate between orthodromic and antidromic conduction.**

Orthodromic conduction is in the direction of physiologic nerve transmission (e.g., toward the spinal cord for orthodromic sensory potentials). Antidromic conduction is in the opposite direction of physiologic nerve transmission (e.g., away from the spinal cord for antidromic sensory potentials).

**What parameters of NCS are routinely evaluated?**

The latency (time from stimulation to response) and amplitude of the responses are measured; the conduction velocity along the nerve may be calculated.

**What findings on NCS are characteristic of primarily demyelinating neuropathies, and why?**

Slowed conduction velocities and prolonged latencies due to demyelination

**What findings on NCS are characteristic of primarily axonal neuropathies, and why?**

Decreased amplitudes due to axonal loss

# 46                Electroencephalography

**What is an electroencephalogram (EEG)?**

A method of recording electrical activity of the brain

**How is it performed?**

Many small metal disks, called electrodes, are placed on the scalp with a conducting paste, in specific locations. The patient can be awake or asleep, and the procedure is not painful.

**What is a contraindication to EEG?**

There are no absolute contraindications, although it may be difficult in some circumstances (e.g., with a noncooperative child)

**What is a recording montage?**

The display of electrical activity, arranged in a logical fashion, to permit interpretation

**In what two common circumstances is EEG useful?**

In evaluation of:
1. Suspected epilepsy
2. Encephalopathy

**What EEG pattern is most commonly associated with metabolic encephalopathy?**

Generalized slowing

**What EEG pattern is classically associated with hepatic encephalopathy?**

Triphasic waves—however, they may occur with almost any metabolic encephalopathy

**Overdose of which drug is most likely to produce an isoelectric EEG?**

Barbiturates

**What EEG pattern is associated with focal structural disease?**

Focal slowing

## EEG AND SEIZURE

**Does a normal EEG exclude the diagnosis of epilepsy?**

No (see Chapter 8)

**Characterize typical EEG changes occurring during a seizure.**

Sudden onset of sharp, rhythmic EEG activity that is distinguishable from the background activity and is of a finite duration

**Characterize three types of epileptiform activity on EEG.**

Spikes (20–70 msec), sharp waves (70–200 msec), or an electrographic seizure.

**Describe a spike wave.**

It would hurt if you sat on it (i.e., a very sharp-pointed deflection that stands out from the background and is often followed by a slow wave). See figure.

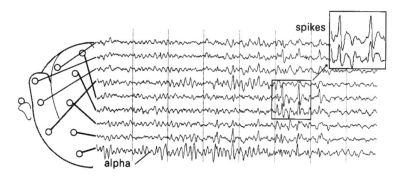

**What is the significance of focal spikes or sharp waves?**

It means there is a focal area of overly excitable (potentially epileptic) cortex.

**What is the significance of generalized spikes or sharp waves?**

The whole brain is overly excitable *or* a focal area of excitability is very rapidly spreading.

**What EEG abnormality is most common in patients with focal seizures?**

Focal sharp waves and spikes

**What EEG abnormality is most common in patients with generalized seizures?**

Generalized sharp waves and spikes

**Compare the terms *focal* and *partial*.**

They have the same meaning.

**How often is the first EEG abnormal in patients with a focal epilepsy?**

About 50% of the time. A second EEG yields a cumulative sensitivity of ~70%.

**What techniques are commonly used to increase the probability of epileptiform activity on EEG?**

Activation procedures include photic stimulation, hyperventilation, sleep, and sleep deprivation.

**What is the only EEG finding absolutely diagnostic of a seizure?**

An electrographic seizure recorded during a typical clinical seizure

**Describe the EEG pattern of absence epilepsy.**

Generalized 3-Hz spike and wave, often provoked by hyperventilation

**What age group is most susceptible to absence seizures?**

Children

# 47

# Evoked Potentials

## VISUAL EVOKED POTENTIALS (VEPs)

**How is a VEP performed?**
A visual pattern is presented to the patient, and the cerebral response is measured by electrodes placed over the occipital region.

**What does the patient look at during a pattern-reversal VEP?**
A television screen displaying a checkerboard pattern that alternates between black and white

**What signal from the occipital cortex is the most reproducible and clinically relevant?**
P100

**VEPs are an extension of which component of the neurologic exam?**
Visual field testing

**In what clinical context is a VEP most useful?**
1. Evaluation of otherwise occult visual pathway lesions (as in possible MS)
2. To determine where a lesion occurs in the visual pathway (i.e., pre- or postchiasmatic)

**Can uncooperative or encephalopathic patients successfully perform pattern-reversal VEPs?**
No. Patients must be able to fix their gaze on the visual stimulus.

## BRAIN STEM AUDITORY-EVOKED POTENTIALS (BAEPs)

**How is a BAEP performed?**
The patient is given an auditory "click" through a headset, and the brain-stem response is measured by electrodes placed on the head.

| | |
|---|---|
| **What are the three most important waves measured during BAEPs?** | Waves I, III, and V |
| **What are their anatomic correlates?** | The exact neural generators are controversial, but wave I originates peripherally, wave III in the lateral pons, and wave V originates in the midbrain. |
| **BAEPs are an extension of which component of the neurologic exam?** | Cranial nerve examination |
| **In what clinical context is a BAEP most useful?** | To evaluate painless hearing loss<br>To rule out an eighth nerve lesion<br>To investigate brain-stem dysfunction<br>To evaluate coma |
| **What makes BAEPs useful in some cases of assessing coma?** | BAEPs remain intact throughout most nonstructural causes of brain-stem dysfunction |

## SOMATOSENSORY EVOKED POTENTIALS (SSEPs)

| | |
|---|---|
| **How are SSEPs performed?** | A peripheral nerve is electrically stimulated, and the response is measured in the proximal peripheral nerve, spinal cord, and cortex by electrodes placed in these areas. |
| **What are the two most common stimulation sites?** | Median nerve (MN) at the wrist and posterior tibial nerve (PTN) at the ankle (see figure) |

**What are the common sites for electrode placement for SSEPs?**

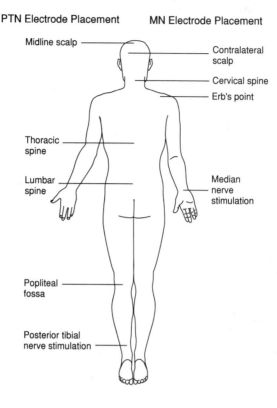

PTN Electrode Placement     MN Electrode Placement

Midline scalp

Contralateral scalp

Cervical spine

Erb's point

Thoracic spine

Lumbar spine

Median nerve stimulation

Popliteal fossa

Posterior tibial nerve stimulation

| | |
|---|---|
| **SSEPs are an extension of which component of the neurologic exam?** | Sensory examination |
| **When are SSEPs indicated?** | To assess level of a lesion causing sensory symptoms<br>To evaluate traumatic myelopathy<br>For intraoperative monitoring during spinal cord surgery to evaluate prognosis in coma |
| **What clinical syndrome is associated with giant SSEP?** | Progressive myoclonic epilepsies |
| **What response occurs in a patient with myelopathy?** | With myelopathy, no signal is detected above the spinal cord. |
| **With a lesion at the cortex?** | With a lesion at the cortex, no signal is detected at the scalp. |
| **What finding indicates a poor prognosis in coma?** | Lack of cortical responses despite the presence of spinal cord responses |

# 48

# Tensilon (Edrophonium) Test

**What is the purpose of a Tensilon test?**

To detect a defect of neuromuscular transmission (e.g., as occurs in myasthenia gravis)

**How is it performed?**

Ten mg of Tensilon are drawn up into a 1 ml syringe. Two mg (0.2 ml) are injected i.v. as a test dose. If no response is seen, the remaining 8 mg are injected. A positive response is transient improvement of weakness (e.g., reduced ptosis).

**What is the mechanism of action?**

Edrophonium briefly inhibits acetylcholine esterase and thereby increases the amount of acetylcholine in the neuromuscular junction.

**What is an important cardiac complication?**

Bradycardia caused by cholinergic parasympathetic stimulation

**How is this side effect prevented or treated?**

Injection of atropine

**What are other side effects?**

Nausea; sweating caused by systemic effects of increased acetylcholine

## Table 48–1. Neurogenetic Reference Table

### (A) Brain Malformations

| Disease | Chromosome(s) | Gene Product(s) |
|---|---|---|
| Holoprosencephaly | 7 | Sonic Hedgehog |
| Schizencephaly | 10 | EMX2 homeobox gene |
| Megalencephaly (Canavan's) | 17 | Aspartoacylase |
| Megalencephaly (Alexander's) | 17 | GFAP |
| X-Linked Lissencephaly (males) | X | Doublecortin |
| Double Cortex Syndrome (females) | X | Doublecortin |
| Miller-Dieker Lissencephaly | 17 | Lis 1 |
| Bilateral Periventricular Nodular Heterotopias | X | Filamen 1 |

### (B) Phakomatoses

| Disease | Chromosome(s) | Gene Product(s) |
|---|---|---|
| Von Hippel-Lindau | 3 | VHL |
| Tuberous Sclerosis | 9; 16 | Hamartin; Tuberin |
| Neurofibromatosis I (Von Recklinghausen's) | 17 | Neurofibromin |
| Neurofibromatosis II | 22 | Merlin (schwannomin) |
| Ataxia Telangiectasia | 11 | ATM |
| Sturge Weber | — (Sporadic) | ? |

### (C) Muscular Dystrophies

| Disease | Chromosome(s) | Gene Product(s) |
|---|---|---|
| Duchenne | X | Dystrophin |
| Becker | X | Dystrophin |
| Myotonic | 19 | Myotonin protein kinase |
| Fascioscapulohumeral | Telomeric 4q | ? |
| Scapuloperoneal | Some with 12 linkage | ? |
| Oculopharyngeal | 14 | PABP2 |
| Limb Girdle (over 10 types) | Multiple | Include caveolin 3, calpain, dysferlin, sarcoglycan, adhalin |
| Emery-Dreifuss | X | Emerin |

## Table 48–1. (*Continued*)

**(D) Neuropathies**

| Disease | Chromosome(s) | Gene Product(s) |
| --- | --- | --- |
| Amyloid Polyneuropathies | 18; 11 | Transthyretin; apolipoprotein A-1 |
| NARP | Mitochondrial | ATPase 6 |
| Charcot-Marie-Tooth forms of HMSN (I, II) | 17; 1; X | PMP22; P0; connexin 32 |
| Dejerine-Sottas form of HMSN (III) | 17 | PMP22 |
| Refsum's Disease form of HMSN (IV) | 10 | Phytanoyl-CoA hydroxylase |
| Tomaculous Neuropathy | 17 | PMP22 |

NARP = Neuropathy, ataxia, retinitis pigmentosa; HMSN = Hereditary motor and sensory neuropathy.

**(E) Movement Disorders**

| Disease | Chromosome(s) | Gene Product(s) |
| --- | --- | --- |
| DRPLA | 12 | Atrophin |
| Huntington's | 4 | Huntingtin |
| Wilson's | 13 | ATP7B copper transporting ATPase |
| Hyperekplexia | 5 | GLRA1 |
| Dystonia | 9; 14; X; Mitochondrial | Torsin A; GTP cyclohydrolase; TIMM8A; ND6 |
| PARK1 (An autosomal dominant form of PD) | 4 | α synuclein |
| PARK2 (An autosomal recessive form of PD) | 6 | parkin |
| PARK3 (An autosomal dominant form of PD) | 2 | ? |
| PARK4 (An autosomal dominant form of PD) | 4 | ? |
| PARK5 (An autosomal dominant form of PD) | 4 | ubiquitin carboxy-terminal dehydrolase (UCH-L1) |

DRPLA = Dentatorubropallidoluysian atrophy;
PD = Parkinson's disease;
? = linkage only.

## Table 48–1. (*Continued*)

### (F) Dementias

| Disease | Chromosome(s) | Gene Product(s) |
|---|---|---|
| Alzheimer's (autosomal dominant forms only) | 21; 14; 1 | Amyloid precursor protein; presenilin 1; presenilin 2 |
| Alzheimer's (increases risk of sporadic forms) | 19 | APOE4 variant of APOE |
| Frontotemporal Dementia with Parkinsonism (autosomal dominant form) | 17 | Tau |
| CADASIL | 19 | Notch3 |
| Jacob-Creutzfeldt (autosomal dominant form) | 20 | PRNP |

CADASIL = Cerebral autosomal dominant arteriopathy with subcortical infarcts and leukoencephalopathy.

### (G) Motor Pathway Degenerations

| Disease | Chromosome(s) | Gene Product(s) |
|---|---|---|
| ALS (Some autosomal dominant forms) | 21 | Copper-zinc superoxide dismutase |
| Hereditary Spastic Paraparesis (recessive form) | 16 | Paraplegin |
| Hereditary Spastic Paraparesis (dominant form) | 2 | Spastin |
| Spinal Muscular Atrophy | 5 | SMN; NAIP |

### (H) Progressive Myoclonic Epilepsies

| Disease Name | OMIM Name | Chromosome | Gene or Product |
|---|---|---|---|
| Unverricht-Lundborg | EPM1 | 21 | Cystatin B |
| Lafora Disease | EPM2 | 6 | Tyrosine phosphatase (Laforin) |
| NCL (Batten's) | CLN3 | 16 | Lysosome protease |
| NCL with Granular Osmiophilic Deposits | CLN1 | 1 | Palmitoyl protein thioesterase |
| Sialidosis Type 1 | — | 6 | Neuraminidase |
| MERRF | — | Mitochondrial | tRNA Lys |
| DRPLA | — | 12 | Ataxin |

OMIM = Online mendelian inheritance in man (www.ncbi.nlm.hih.gov/omim/);

NCL = Neuronal ceroid lipofuscinosis; MERRF = Myoclonic epilepsy and ragged red fiber disease; DRPLA = Dentatorubropallidoluysian atrophy.

## Table 48–1. (*Continued*)

### (I) Mitochondrial DNA Diseases

| Disease | Mutation(s) | Gene(s) |
|---------|-------------|---------|
| Mitochondrial Encephalopathy, Lactic Acidosis, and Stroke (MELAS) | A3243G; T3271C | tRNA LEU (UUR) |
| Myoclonic Epilepsy and Ragged Red Fiber Disease (MERRF) | A8344G; T8356C | tRNA Lys |
| Kearns Sayre Chronic Progressive External Opthalmoplegia | Deletions; A3243G | Missing genes; tRNA LEU (UUR) |
| Neuropathy, Ataxia, Retinitis Pigmentosa (NARP) | T8993G | ATPase 6 |
| Maternally Inherited Leigh's Disease | T8993G | ATPase 6 |
| Leber's Hereditary Optic Neuropathy | Multiple | Many in NADH dehydrogenase genes; one in the cytochrome B gene |

### (J) Type I Trinucleotide Repeat Disorders (repeats are translated*)

| Disease | Chromosome | Gene | Repeat | Normal Length | Disease Length |
|---------|-----------|------|--------|--------------|---------------|
| Huntington's | 4 | Huntingtin | CAG | 10–34 | 37–121 |
| DRPLA | 12 | Atrophin | CAG | 7–34 | 49–83 |
| SCA1 | 6 | Ataxin 1 | CAG | 6–44 | 42–83 |
| SCA2 | 12 | Ataxin 2 | CAG | 15–32 | 35–77 |
| SCA3/MJD | 14 | Ataxin 3/MJD1 | CAG | 12–39 | 66–84 |
| SCA6 | 19 | Calcium channel | CAG | 3–17 | 21–30 |
| SCA7 | 3 | Ataxin 7 | CAG | 4–35 | 38–200 |
| SCA12 | 5 | Ataxin 12 | CAG | <29 | 66–78 |
| Kennedy's | X | Androgen receptor | CAG | 11–33 | 40–66 |

DRPLA = dentatorubropallidoluysian atrophy; SCA = spinocerebellar atrophy; MJD = Machado Joseph disease.

* The expansion gets converted into a polyglutamine amino acid stretch in the protein.

**Table 48–1. (Continued)**

**(K) Type II Triple Repeat Disorders (repeats are not translated\*)**

| Disease | Chromosome | Gene | Repeat | Normal Length | Disease Length |
|---------|-----------|------|--------|---------------|----------------|
| FRAX-A | X | FMR-1 | CGG | 6–54 | 200–1500 |
| FRAX-E | X | FMR-2 | CCG | 6–25 | 200–1000 |
| Myotonic Dystrophy | 19 | Myotonin protein kinase | CTG | 5–37 | 200–3000 |
| SCA8 | 13 | — | CTG | 16–91 | 107–127 |
| Freidreich's Ataxia | 9 | Frataxin | GAA | 7–40 | 81–1700 |

FRAX = fragile X syndrome; SCA = spinocerebellar atrophy.

\* The repeat is in an intron or untranslated region and does not cause placement of amino acids into the protein; problems may arise from structural RNA changes due to very long nucleotide expansions.

**(L) Channelopathies**

| Disease | Ion Channel | Chromosome | Gene |
|---------|-------------|------------|------|
| Hyperkalemic Periodic Paralysis | Sodium | 17 | SCN4 |
| Paramyotonia Congenita (von Eulenberg) | Sodium | 17 | SCN4 |
| Malignant Hypothermia (some) | Sodium | 17 | SCN4 |
| Hypokalemic Periodic Paralysis (rare forms) | Sodium | 17 | SCN4 |
| Generalized Epilepsy with Febrile Seizures (Type 1) | Sodium | 19 | SCN1B |
| Generalized Epilepsy with Febrile Seizures (Type 2) | Sodium | 2 | SCN1A |
| Hypokalemic Periodic Paralysis (most forms) | Calcium | 1 | CACNAIS (CACNL1A3) |
| Spinocerebellar Ataxia Type 6 | Calcium | 19 | CACNA1A (CACNL1A4) |
| Some Generalized Epilepsy | Calcium | 2 | CACNB4 |
| Hypokalemic Periodic Paralysis (rare forms) | Potassium | 11 | KCNE3 |
| Benign Familial Neonatal Convulsions (EBN1) | Potassium | 20 | KCNQ2 |
| Benign Familial Neonatal Convulsions (EBN2) | Potassium | 8 | KCNQ3 |
| Episodic Ataxia Type 1 | Potassium | 12 | KCNA1 |
| Kinesiogenic Choreoathetosis with Episodic Ataxia and Spasticity; DYT9 | Potassium | 1 | KCNA3 (?) |
| Becker Myotonia Congenita | Chloride | 7 | CLCN1 |
| Thomsen Myotonia Congenita | Chloride | 7 | CLCN1 |

# Index

Note: Page numbers in *italics* indicate illustrations; those followed by t indicate tables.